teach® yourself

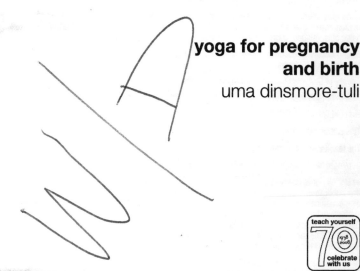

yoga for pregnancy and birth
uma dinsmore-tuli

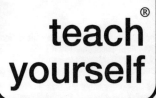

teach yourself
70
1938 2008
celebrate with us

Launched in 1938, the **teach yourself** series grew rapidly in response to the world's wartime needs. Loved and trusted by over 50 million readers, the series has continued to respond to society's changing interests and passions and now, 70 years on, includes over 500 titles, from Arabic and Beekeeping to Yoga and Zulu. What would you like to learn?

be where you want to be with **teach yourself**

For UK order enquiries: please contact Bookpoint Ltd, 130 Milton Park, Abingdon, Oxon, OX14 4SB. Telephone: +44 (0) 1235 827720. Fax: +44 (0) 1235 400454. Lines are open 09.00–17.00, Monday to Saturday, with a 24-hour message answering service. Details about our titles and how to order are available at www.teachyourself.co.uk.

For USA order enquiries: please contact McGraw-Hill Customer Services, PO Box 545, Blacklick, OH 43004-0545, USA. Telephone: 1-800-722-4726. Fax: 1-614-755-5645.

For Canada order enquiries: please contact McGraw-Hill Ryerson Ltd, 300 Water St, Whitby, Ontario L1N 9B6, Canada. Telephone: 905 430 5000. Fax: 905 430 5020.

Long renowned as the authoritative source for self-guided learning – with more than 50 million copies sold worldwide – the **teach yourself** series includes over 500 titles in the fields of languages, crafts, hobbies, business, computing and education.

British Library Cataloguing in Publication Data: a catalogue record for this title is available from the British Library.

Library of Congress Catalog Card Number: on file.

First published in UK 2008 by Hodder Education, 338 Euston Road, London, NW1 3BH.

First published in US 2008 by The McGraw-Hill Companies, Inc.

This edition published 2008.

The **teach yourself** name is a registered trade mark of Hodder Headline.

Typeset by Transet Limited, Coventry, England.
Printed in Great Britain for Hodder Education, a division of Hodder Headline, an Hachette Livre UK Company, 338 Euston Road, London, NW1 3BH, by Cox & Wyman Ltd, Reading, Berkshire.

The publisher has used its best endeavours to ensure that the URLs for external websites referred to in this book are correct and active at the time of going to press. However, the publisher and the author have no responsibility for the websites and can make no guarantee that a site will remain live or that the content will remain relevant, decent or appropriate.

Hachette's policy is to use papers that are natural, renewable and recyclable products and made from wood grown in sustainable forests. The logging and manufacturing processes are expected to conform to the environmental regulations of the country of origin.

Impression number   10 9 8 7 6 5 4 3 2 1
Year   2012 2011 2010 2009 2008

contents

Summary of routines for specific needs

Health promotion

- For high vitality days: Sun salutation modification, p. 177.
- For quieter, or medium vitality days: Moon sequence, p. 178.
- For days when you are feeling strong and vigorous: Standing flow, p. 180.
- For quieter days when you feel heavier but require an energy boost: Earthed seated flow, p. 181.
- Heart-focused practice for comfort and healing of mother and baby, p. 189.
- Earth-focused practice for stability and security, p. 190.

Healing sequences for relief from pain or discomfort

- To ease and prevent lower back pain, p. 183.
- For prevention and management of pelvic pain and instability (pubis symphysis dysfunction and sacroiliac pain), p. 184.
- For relief of heartburn and indigestion, and to free space in the upper back, p. 185.
- To relieve breathlessness, p. 186.
- To ease tenderness of swollen ankles and/or wrist stiffness, p. 187.
- For exhaustion, p. 188.

Yoga suggestions for birth

- Pre labour, p. 198.
- Established first stage: thinning and opening, p. 200.
- Second stage: birthing the baby, p. 204.
- Third stage: birthing the placenta, p. 208.

Yoga programmes for post-natal recovery

- Nurture: for immediately after birth and up to eight weeks, or whenever you feel more tired than usual, p. 221.
- Stabilize: from four to six weeks after birth, p. 222.
- Restore vitality: at 8–12 weeks, or whenever you have more energy, p. 223.

audio CD contents

The tracks on the audio CD are sample practices from Sitaram Partnership's range of audio CDs (see Taking it further). Written instructions for each track are found on the pages indicated.

Track 1

Full yogic breath/breath of life, including Circle of breath (From *Mother's Breath* CD 1): p. 13–16

Track 2

Ujjayi breath (From *Yogabirth 1*): p. 16

Track 3

Golden thread exhalation (From *Yogabirth 1*): p. 18

Track 4

Peaks and valleys/Ocean waves breath (From *Mother's Breath* CD 2): p. 202

Track 5

Yoga nidra/Baby bond (From *Yogabirth 1*): p. 166–8

Track 6

Inner silence/Feeding meditation (From *Yogababies*): p. 168–70

Track 7

Purnamada/Chant for abundance and acceptance (From *Mother's Breath* CD 3): p. 175

acknowledgements

All the practices in this book have been tried and tested in Sitaram yoga classes since 1997. I am thankful to all of our pregnant students whose positive feedback has developed this approach to pregnancy yoga. I am especially grateful to the midwifery departments of St Thomas's and King's College Hospitals for providing practical support for these classes. In particular I would like to thank Katie Yiannouzis, Head of Midwifery at King's College Hospital, and Geraldine Joyce, Head of Midwifery at St Thomas's Hospital. The practical encouragement that both Katie and Geraldine have given to these classes, by providing teaching venues in their respective hospitals, has made the benefits of yoga more widely available to many women in London.

I am thankful to midwife Teresa Arias (South London Independent Midwives) and yoga teacher Frankie Duggan for their valuable advice on Chapter 08 and to Natasha Rhoden, pregnant with baby Ocean, for modelling many of the poses. Thanks also to Mohini Chatlani for permission to include the Victory pose of the fierce goddess and Lord of the Dance sequence from her book *Yogaflows;* Sofya Ansari (yoga teacher and ayurvedic practitioner) for permission to include the Heart-womb breath and Sufi head tilt mudra from her forthcoming book *Blooming Mother, Blissful Baby*; and Mukunda Stiles for permission to include the Joint freeing series from *Structural Yoga Therapy*.

Thanks to the team at Hodder Education for their skilful support: to Victoria Roddam for inviting me to write the book, and to Jenny Organ for making it all happen.

Gratitude and appreciation to the Goenka and Poddar households in Kolkata for generous hospitality during the gestation of the book, and Swami Satyasangananda and Paramahamsa Satyananda for enabling my family to enjoy the peace of Rikhia when I was writing the first draft. This book was written during my pregnancy with Rajakumari Prayaag Eileen Dinsmore-Tuli, my third child. Her guiding presence shaped the project from beginning to end. Thank you.

preface

I am delighted that pregnancy yoga classes are provided here on site at King's by Sitaram Partnership because it gives women the impression that we are broad-minded and flexible, and that we do not only support a medical model of care, which may make our service appeal to more women. I am very happy that they can attend yoga classes on site where they may become more comfortable as their pregnancies progress and where the hospital may become less of a scary environment.

My observations of women in labour, after they attend pregnancy yoga classes, are that they can focus more on the work they have to do and remain calm and feel in control. For some there has been a remarkable journey during pregnancy from being fearful of labour to managing the process very well.

Katie Yiannouzis
Head of Midwifery, King's College Hospital,
London SE5

introduction

This mother's guide to yoga for spirit, mind and body includes breath, relaxation, movement and meditations for every stage of pregnancy, including labour, birth and post-natal recovery. It also includes an audio CD.

Who is this book for?

Teach Yourself Yoga for Pregnancy and Birth provides clear guidance for safe and enjoyable practice of all aspects of yoga in pregnancy. Its intention is to enable you to benefit from suitable yoga practices without the need of a teacher. However, it may also serve as a useful companion and support for pregnant women already attending yoga classes, and for yoga teachers whose students are pregnant. Expectant mothers with a pre-pregnancy yoga practice may also find that the book provides refreshing new perspectives on yoga. Many of the practices, particularly those in Chapters 08 and 09, which relate directly to the application of yoga during birth and post-natal recovery, may be of interest to midwives and other health professionals who care for pregnant women.

What kind of yoga can I learn from this book?

Because some of the most popular forms of yoga in the West are those with a strong emphasis upon its physical aspects, there is a common misperception that yoga is primarily a series of physical exercises. There is no doubt that yoga certainly brings many benefits to the physical body, improving general health and boosting vitality, promoting strength, and encouraging a full range of movement, whilst supporting the effective functioning of every system of the body. But this aspect is only a tiny part of what it has to offer. The approach presented here is holistic. Physical practice is one part of a broader system that places equal emphasis upon emotional, energetic and spiritual experience. A comprehensive practice of yoga, such as that presented here, includes inner and outer attitudes and observances (yama and niyama), breath practices (pranayama), sensory integration (pratyahara), energy locks (bandha), symbolic gesture (mudra), sound work (nada and mantra), deep relaxation and meditation as well as postures (asana).

Following an outline of the purpose of yoga and its relevance to pregnancy and birth (Chapter 01), practical instructions begin with four primary breath awareness practices (Chapter 02). It is necessary to gain basic familiarity with these core breaths before moving on to other techniques, because everything else that follows rests on their foundation.

After the core breaths, each chapter focuses upon a discrete but related 'layer' of human experience, working from the physical body (Chapter 03), through the experience of the energy field (Chapter 04), to access emotional, mental and spiritual experiences (Chapters 05, 06 and 07) that are all part of a full spectrum of yoga practice.

Chapters 03 to 07 are organized according to the yoga system of 'five bodies'. Thus, practices for the physical body are explored as a manifestation of the earth element, those for the energy field are understood as an expression of the element water, whilst the experiences of emotional life and the insights of wisdom are considered in relation to the elements air and ether. Chapter 07 describes how an integrated practice can connect with the experience of pure joy which exists beyond these elements. Chapters 08 and 09 are about yoga for birth and post-natal recovery.

How to use this book and audio CD

There are many ways to use this book. For a complete picture of what yoga has to offer at this time, it is best to read the whole book, although not necessarily in the order in which it is presented. For example, if your main interest is in yoga for birth (Chapter 07), or for coping with the intense emotional life of pregnancy (Chapter 04), then it's wisest to turn to the chapter which deals directly with your concern. If you are experiencing particular difficulties or challenges and are seeking yoga remedies and preventions, or are hunting for the instructions to a particular yoga practice, then it is simplest to consult the index to locate the technique/s specifically recommended in that instance.

In the absence of a particularly pressing concern or interest, then the wisest approach is to work with the practical suggestions for each aspect of experience, beginning with the chapter whose focus seems most vivid to you right now. Follow the suggestions to ensure the practice is tailored appropriately to your present stage of pregnancy, and then expand your reading and practice to take on board the focus of the other chapters as you gain confidence and familiarity with the practices you have learnt. Sample holistic programmes, including elements from all aspects of practice, are provided in Chapter 07. These sample programmes enable you to build an appropriate and enjoyable home practice for your journey through pregnancy.

The tracks on the audio CD are fully integrated with the written instructions in each chapter. As each practice is introduced in the text, you are given references to the relevant audio track. In the first place, it is always best to read through the instructions prior to following the audio track, but once you are familiar with the practice then it is easier to close your eyes and listen to the audio instruction. In order to deepen your experience and understanding of the practices, written and audio texts offer slightly different perspectives on the same techniques. In Chapter 02, for example, the written summaries for three of the essential core breaths (pp. 10–19) are expanded upon by the audio guidance in tracks 1–3 on the CD, whilst in Chapter 06, a full audio practice of yoga nidra (track 5) is supplemented by a written account of the structure and framework of the technique (p. 166).

Once you are familiar with both the written and audio instructions for each of the practices on the CD, then it is also possible (and enjoyable) to listen to the whole CD all the way through, as it provides a complete, hour-long practice of breath and awareness. Alternatively, choose the practices that best suit your needs at a particular time, and just listen to one or two tracks. For example, listening to track 1 and track 5 (Full yogic breath followed by yoga nidra) takes about 25 minutes and provides an effective programme of relaxation suitable for anytime when you need to boost your energy and rest deeply.

All the audio tracks promote a state of deep relaxation, so please do not listen to the CD whilst you are driving, or operating machinery.

Where do the practices come from?

The practices described in this book offer a practical, safe and holistic approach to yoga for pregnancy and birth that has been tried and tested by thousands of women. Principally the method develops from yoga therapy, the main concern of which is to adapt the practice of yoga to the needs of the individual. Unless otherwise identified in the texts and references, the majority of the practices in this book, including postures, deep relaxation and some of the breath practices are from the Satyananda (Bihar School) system of yoga, and most are also informed by guidelines for safe practice established by Mukunda Stiles' Structural Yoga Therapy™. The principles of asana modification and transitional moves for pregnancy, which inform some poses presented in Chapter 03 and are the basis of the Birthing breath in Chapter 08, both stem from the approach pioneered by Françoise Freedman, founder of the Birthlight Trust. Most of the sound, hand gesture and flowing posture sequences are a creative synthesis of existing practices.

Beyond these roots, this approach to pregnancy yoga is informed by the understanding gained from teaching yoga to pregnant women since 1996 and training pregnancy yoga teachers since 2000. These activities have their original inspiration in my own experiences as a pregnant woman practising yoga.

Every pregnancy is unique, and each woman finds her own way through her journey. With each of my three pregnancies, I have found yoga to be of great assistance, but only in so far as it was appropriate to the specific needs of that pregnancy. For example, during the first pregnancy, when I was training as a yoga therapist, and had already been practicing yoga for five years, I conducted a comparative study to sample different approaches to pregnancy yoga teaching. Having explored what was on offer (more details of classes in Taking it further), I learnt to make some helpful adaptations to the yoga systems I was using at the time. Mostly I stuck to my existing practice, and sailed through pregnancy and birth with few difficulties at a physical level, but found sound work and deep relaxation (yoga nidra) to be invaluable in the management of the turbulent emotional life of pregnancy. I also experienced, during the process of that first labour, the gift of a profoundly powerful breath practice that transformed my ability to accept and manage physical and emotional pain. My encounter with this practice, later called the Golden thread breath (p. 18), changed my approach to teaching pregnancy yoga.

During a second pregnancy, two years later, I was (like many women) so exhausted that the main suitable practices were quieter sitting meditations with pranayama and deep relaxation.

Writing this book during a third pregnancy, seven years later than the first, it is the deep support of restorative yoga and the creative synthesis of sound, hand gesture (mudra) and flowing movement (such as those described in Chapter 07) that provide most nourishment.

These contrasting experiences of the function of different forms of yoga during pregnancy and birth demonstrate how yoga may be of benefit to pregnant students. In addition to the diverse experience of my own three pregnancies, I have been privileged to share the experiences of thousands of students who have attended Sitaram's pregnancy and birth yoga programme since 1997. Some of these women came to yoga during pregnancy because they had an existing practice and were seeking to expand or adapt it to accommodate the changes of pregnancy, but many more of the students had never done yoga before they became pregnant. It is these women who have tried, tested and testified to the practical benefit of the techniques in *Teach Yourself Yoga for Pregnancy and Birth*. The voices of these women speak directly in personal accounts accompanying the instructions for many practices in the book.

Can you really teach yourself yoga?

It is customary at the start of any text about yoga for the author to sound a cautionary note about the very concept of learning yoga from a book. This caution becomes especially necessary when the title of the book clearly states that the book is intended to enable you to 'teach yourself' yoga. Some context clarifies the reality of this option. All the techniques presented in *Teach Yourself Yoga for Pregnancy and Birth* are drawn from the great river of yoga practice that has been flowing out of India for the past 3,000 years. The river's course has become astonishingly wide and long, with many tributaries, off-shoots and backwaters, so that now its waters irrigate much of the planet, with gifted teachers, practitioners and trainers of yoga all over the world. During its long history, the traditional way for yoga to be taught is to be passed on from teacher to student, in an unbroken lineage of personal instruction, with the teacher tailoring the teachings to meet the specific needs of the individual student. This is no doubt the very best way to learn yoga, and no book could ever replace a teacher's personal guidance, nor offer the refined adjustments and modifications that a skilled instructor can provide.

If there is any possibility to supplement the instructions in this book by personal connection with an experienced teacher trained in yoga for pregnancy (preferably in a small group), then I would urge you to do so, especially if you have any health concerns. The number of teachers trained to teach yoga suited to pregnant women is rapidly increasing, and details of how to find a teacher are provided in Taking it further. Yoga classes specifically for pregnant women tend to be friendly, informal and accessible to women who have never done yoga before.

Case study – Lucy

Lucy first began to practise yoga during her first pregnancy with her daughter Sophie and her experience is very typical: 'I loved it. It gave me some invaluable 'time out' each week in a busy life to focus on me and my growing baby and let me feel very special. The classes also provided me with vital tips on taking care of myself throughout pregnancy and labour – information that I didn't get in any other antenatal classes or books. Not only that, but it gave me a great chance to meet some other mothers-to-be who have since become friends.'

The inner teacher

Even within yoga traditions that insist the authentic transmission of yoga can occur only through a teacher–student lineage, there is recognition of the sound guidance that comes from an individual's inner teacher. The greatest learning and most valuable benefits of yoga practice are understood in all traditions to come not from what is learnt in a class, but from what the student learns when she practises by herself. It is in these periods of 'self practice' that the guiding voice of the inner teacher can be heard most clearly and directly. This inner teacher does not rely upon external instruction, but seeks to align the student with the greatest good which may be achieved through their practice of yoga. Hearing the guidance of the inner teacher can be as simple as following the signals given by the body to always move and breathe in the manner which creates the deepest sense of comfort and peace. In this way, even in the absence of the personal instruction from a teacher, it is perfectly possible to gain great benefit from the practice of yoga.

The intention of *Teach Yourself Yoga for Pregnancy and Birth* is to provide you with sufficient understanding to follow the guidance of your own inner teacher. It includes not only the instructions for each practice, but also explanations and tips to alert you to the aims and expected effects of each technique. In this way, the book provides you with a firm foundation from which to practise with confidence those elements of yoga that are most appropriate and beneficial for you. This confidence comes from the recognition that the wisest form of practice is that in which the student follows the guidance of the inner teacher, and that guidance always comes from a feeling of heart. The wisest approach to yoga, as to life, is to preface all action with acknowledgment of one's inner guide:

> With great respect and love, I honour my heart, my inner teacher.
>
> Mukunda Stiles, *Structural Yoga Therapy*

dedication

For my dad, Jim Moore, who taught me some very important things, especially to follow my heart.

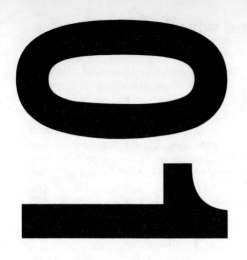

01

yoga and pregnancy: natural partners

In this chapter you will learn:
- about the benefits of yoga throughout pregnancy and after
- about the five yoga bodies
- about the practicalities for your yoga practice.

What is yoga and why do it in pregnancy?

Yoga is an ancient, complete and effective system of self-care and spiritual development. Both its foundation and its ultimate aim are an experience of 'union' or sense of harmony between the individual being and the vital lifeforce that animates the universe in which we live. The techniques of yoga are a refined and subtle technology of psycho-spiritual transformation enacted through the body. Yet they are often simple to learn and accessible to everybody. When you embark on a yoga journey, the act of practising yoga opens the possibility for transformation, which often manifests in a sense of improved well-being, altered perspectives, increased vitality and greater clarity of understanding. The self-care aspect of yoga practice promotes clearer awareness and understanding of your own physical needs, and provides you with tools to meet these needs. The practice of yoga enables you to enjoy higher energy levels, improved immunity, more restful sleep, better digestion, greater range of movement, a stronger body and a more balanced outlook on life. Beginning a journey of yoga is the start of a commitment to self-transformation that begins with the encouraging benefits of evidently improved general health.

When you embark on the journey of pregnancy and birth, you enter a time of major life change, which also has the capacity to transform your way of being at every level. Pregnancy is a period of daily change in the physical bodies of mother and unborn child, accompanied by constant shifting experiences of energy, vitality and exhaustion. Yoga is of great practical assistance during this time, because its techniques of breath, movement, meditation and relaxation support your adaptation to pregnancy with ease and comfort. A sensitive and appropriate practice of yoga in pregnancy responds to the physical changes and any minor ailments of pregnancy with yoga remedies and preventives that can help you to experience pregnancy as a special state of health, a time of well-being and delight.

But yoga is much more than just a helpful practical companion to support the physical aspect of the journey towards motherhood. At every step of the way, yoga's underlying philosophy of 'union' provides a framework of understanding that enables the pregnant traveller to adapt with grace and acceptance to deep levels of emotional, energetic and spiritual change. Pregnancy is a time of heightened mental and emotional experience, characterized by transitions through a broad spectrum of feelings and thought processes. The yoga systems of breath awareness, deep relaxation, visualizations and meditations provide you with effective ways to process the sometimes overwhelming shifts of mood, attitude and perceptions that measure out the journey towards motherhood. Simple but profound techniques of breath awareness and hand gesture, together with deep relaxation and mantra (sound work) can equip you to navigate a safe passage through pregnancy and birth to your own birth as a mother.

During pregnancy the powerful challenges of these many physical, energetic and emotional transformations can lead women to access the intuitive wisdom in which the system of yoga is grounded. This wisdom can be brought to consciousness through the experiences of your physical body, vitality, thoughts and feelings. As you nurture and nourish the unborn child, the pregnant body becomes a vivid physical embodiment of unconditional love, a micro-universe of generous abundance, protecting and feeding the growing child within.

From the yoga perspective, to be pregnant is to be in this state of 'union' every second of each day. This is why pregnant women make great yoga students. Yoga and pregnancy are very natural partners. In pregnancy a woman is naturally, psycho-biologically and hormonally hardwired to experience the state of 'union' to which yoga leads. The practice of yoga brings conscious awareness to this natural tendency during pregnancy, and becoming conscious of messages from the physical body can lead to an uncovering of intuitive wisdom. Through this intuitive wisdom comes a profound connection with the joyous pulse that powers the universe, and this can help women to encounter the adventure of mothering in a spirit of acceptance and joy.

The 'five yoga bodies' and their elements

Yoga offers a clear model for understanding the interplay between the physical world, the energy that animates it, and the cosmic perspective of harmonious unity with the life force. This model can be especially helpful to understand during pregnancy, when boundaries between different levels of experience become blurred, and when there is heightened perception at every level of being.

The yoga understanding is that we inhabit not one but five bodies. The physical body is both surrounded and pervaded by energy. Conscious attention to the breath provides the link between our physical experience and the energy which determines the nature of that physical experience. The breath is the bridge between the physical and the energetic. This bridge is the connection between our flesh and blood and our feelings, our energetic sphere of influence in the world. The existence of this bridge and the links between the other bodies or 'sheaths of existence' (*koshas*) is described in the *Taittiriya Upanishad* (book two, verses 8–9, 21), the third among the earliest of the 3,000-year-old Upanishads from which the yoga stream of philosophy flows.

In yoga the flesh and blood body is called *annamaya kosha* – *anna* meaning food, *maya* meaning full of, or made from, and *kosha* meaning sheath, or layer. So, the flesh and blood body is our physical manifestation, built from food. Without our energy to animate this 'food body', it is lifeless. There is another body, or another 'layer' of experience animating the physical. In yoga this is called the *pranamaya kosha* – *prana* meaning life force, *maya* meaning full of, and *kosha* meaning layer or sheath. It is this energy body which we feel pervading and surrounding our physical body.

In addition to these two bodies – the physical and the energy bodies – the *Taittiriya Upanishad* and other yogic texts set out three further layers of existence, or *koshas*. Deeper than the energy field of *prana* comes the body of the emotional and mental responses, our likes, dislikes, opinions and reactions. This is called the *manomaya kosha*, or the layer of the mind. Then comes the *vijnanomaya kosha*, or the layer of existence where we access a more intuitive wisdom that comes from a place beyond the mind of the previous *kosha*. The last of the five is *anandamaya kosha*, or the bliss body, at which level the individual distinctions of the previous four bodies melt away, and there is an experience of harmonious connection.

Although the Sanskrit terminology may seem disconnected from everyday experience, in practical terms, this descriptive framework of understanding clearly and helpfully explains some of the common experiences of pregnancy, birthing and motherhood. The shift in levels of awareness from one layer of these five yogic bodies to the next helps to explain the relationship between, for example, our state of mind, and the postures and sensations of the physical body. When you stand well grounded, with a comfortable carrying position for your unborn child, when your chest is free and open, your head lifted and neck long, it is easier to feel open-hearted, balanced and giving.

If the needs of the physical body (annamaya kosha) are attended to, for example if you are well fed and rested, and supported in a comfortable position, then you can access a deeper, more nourishing breath that boosts your energy levels (pranamaya kosha). It also helps you to observe the chattering of the mind (manomaya kosha) with some equanimity and to access aspects of higher wisdom (vijnanomaya kosha) that help you to connect with an intrinsic state of peace and bliss (anandamaya).

The three trimesters of pregnancy

The journey of pregnancy is often divided into three stages: the first 16 weeks, the period from 16 to about 30 weeks, and the later weeks of pregnancy leading up to the birth. Experiences across each stage are often markedly different, with the first period marked by deep exhaustion, the middle period affording a more stable physical experience of pregnancy, and the last period presenting challenges associated with greater weight and erratic energy levels. The beauty of a holistic yoga practice is that it offers appropriate practices for each and every stage: nourishing breath and restorative work are more appropriate for the opening part of the journey; more active physical and breath work are suited to the middle stage; and a range of integrated practices can help in the last weeks of pregnancy to prepare for birth with confidence. What may be appropriate at one stage may be uncomfortable in another, so throughout this book, suitable modifications and adjustments are given where necessary.

Labour and birth to postpartum

For many pregnant women, especially those expecting their first baby, it is hard to see beyond the birth of the baby, which marks the end of pregnancy. But of course, the birth of the baby is just the beginning of another, much longer, journey of motherhood. Yoga practice can provide a sense of continuity between pregnancy, birth and mothering. The confidence and calm fostered through physical, emotional and energetic practices during pregnancy not only prepares you to cope as well as you can with the experience of labour and birth, but it also provides for sensitive and effective post-natal recovery and offers practical ways to develop the bond that was established in pregnancy with the unborn child. At every level, physical, mental, emotional and spiritual, yoga provides practical support through some of the most demanding and rewarding periods of a women's life cycle.

Time, place and equipment for yoga practice

Traditionally, yoga asanas (postures) are practised in the mornings before breakfast, or in the evenings before eating. The poses can also be practised at other times, but the usual advice is to wait two or three hours after eating before doing asanas. During pregnancy, when energy levels and blood sugar shifts can be volatile, and nausea, faintness or exhaustion can be signs of hunger, it is wisest to bend these rules a little. The practices offered in this book are gentle enough that there is no harm in having a light snack (for example fruits, toast or a cereal bar) before practice if you feel you need an energy boost, and it is sensible to have water to drink as needed. In fact, it is wiser to attend to signs of hunger and thirst than it is to stick rigidly to the yoga 'rules' and discover you feel faint and wobbly part way through your practice.

Whilst it is ideal to have a room set aside exclusively for yoga, this is not a realistic option for most women. A corner or strip of floor does the job. What is needed is somewhere clean, comfortably warm and uncluttered enough for you to move without coming into contact with walls or furniture. It doesn't need to be a big space, just enough room to stretch out. A small expanse of free wall space can also be useful for some of the poses.

Many forms of yoga practice require no props. For any standing postures and for flowing sequences you will need a mat that does not slip, but if you are mostly doing floor-based practices then a blanket or rug works just as well. To accommodate the special needs of the pregnant body, a few key props are needed:

- 3–4 pillows or cushions to support restorative poses,
- 2–3 yoga blocks or firm cushions for sitting,
- a blanket for cover in relaxation and meditation, and to roll up for support in other practices.

Further props are not crucial, but can be helpful additions for certain practices. In order of usefulness, the extra props you may need are:

- a bolster to support sitting and lying poses (this can be improvised from rolled blankets),
- birthing ball (also called Swiss or fit balls) for sitting-based poses,
- straight backed chair,
- bean bag, for resting poses,
- eye bag or light scarf to cover the eyes during relaxations,
- belt or scarf to assist with some shoulder-opening practices.

All the above props are available from Yogamatters (see details on p. 231). A final practical point to remember before starting your practice is that the bladder is both more relaxed and also compressed in early and late pregnancy, whilst the kidneys are working harder to excrete for two. Don't be surprised if you need to pass water once or twice during your yoga practice. Minimize disruption by choosing a practice place with easy access to the bathroom, and make your visits at scheduled breaks, for example in between changes in base position, or before you begin a relaxation practice.

02

the essence of yoga in practice

In this chapter you will learn:
- why breath awareness is the heart of yoga
- how to do the four core breaths
- top tips for each breath.

Heart of yoga

The primary value of yoga during pregnancy and birth is to encourage conscious attention of the natural movement of the breath. This is the single most useful practice which yoga has to offer at any time of life, but is a treasure during pregnancy and birth.

By learning to acknowledge the naturally occurring rhythms of breath (Circle of breath), learning to breathe fully (Full yogic breath) and then learning to use the breath to release (Golden thread exhalation) and to slow physical rhythms (Ujjayi breath), you can acquire a heightened awareness of the needs of body, mind and spirit.

Breathing effectively is vital to well-being in general. If you want to increase your energy levels, then understanding how to breathe fully is the first step. If you want to improve your immunity, optimize your ability to concentrate, manage pain, or simply enjoy more deeply restorative sleep, then yoga breathing is a very helpful tool. With a full and easy breath, the physical body is refreshed, cleansed, nourished and restored. Stress levels drop, vitality increases, and emotional and mental life is more readily balanced. Breathing well is the first step towards living well, and the techniques in this chapter are the essential preliminaries for all good yoga breathing.

Evidently, whenever you make time to do any conscious breath practice during pregnancy, then you are breathing not just for you but also for your baby. Although the benefits of yoga for the mother during pregnancy are widely discussed, it is not often pointed out that the practice of pregnancy yoga, and especially of pranayama (breath and energy practices), builds a bond with the unborn baby. Babies tune in to the rhythm of their mother's breath. They know when you are taking time to relax. Practising yoga together in this way establishes the basis of a relationship with the baby once he or she is born. Babies who have experienced yoga in their mother's womb already recognize relaxed breath patterns, and readily respond to all the sounds and movements of the practices. This recognition of the rhythm and sound of breath can be invaluable in the immediate post-natal period when you and your baby are getting to know each other.

Even if you have never brought conscious attention to your breath, or you have developed restrictive breathing habits, these simple core breaths can make an immediate and welcome difference.

Case study – Marie

I'd never done yoga before I took my first class at 29 weeks pregnant, and what struck me immediately was how beneficial it was for my breathing. I've never been good at breathing deeply, and am prone to panic attacks, but as I learned the Golden thread breathing techniques (p. 18) I discovered that I could, for the first time, fill my lungs without effort. My husband, having spent years listening to my forced, shallow breaths and trying to encourage me to relax, was startled at the change. The benefits of the new breathing habits were dramatic, and continued right through the rest of my pregnancy, birth and into the post-natal period. I found I could relax, and move more easily, and that the newer, fuller breaths changed my mental outlook and boosted my energy.

Preparation and tips for the four core breaths

The core breaths heighten mental and bodily awareness, and help you to slow down; as such these breaths form the foundation for all other practices in this book. Even more crucially they can be used in every day life to promote equanimity, ease and self-confidence. They are also the basis of pain management approaches for labour and birth (p. 192).

To practise these breaths, choose a comfortable and appropriate resting position from those described at the start of the next chapter. When you are first learning the practices, it is often best to begin by lying down, but once you are familiar with them, then they can be done in any posture, even on the move. To settle into the relaxed state necessary for all the breaths, let yourself yawn a few times before you start and close your eyes.

Instructions for these breaths are on tracks 1–3 of the audio CD. It can be easiest to listen to the audio instructions when you begin to learn the breaths, but it is helpful to follow the breath as you read the written instructions before listening to the CD. All of these breaths can be comfortably maintained for long periods of time, but at the outset just aim for five minutes each. When you come to the end of the time you wish to practise, take the mental awareness gently away from the breath, and back to the position in which you are lying or sitting. Breathe in, yawn, stretch and open your eyes.

Circle of breath – the rhythmic breath cycle

The Circle of breath brings clarity of awareness to the rhythms of the natural breath cycle. All of the subsequent core breaths rest upon familiarity with this practice. There is no separate audio track for this breath, since it is best practised at your own pace, reading the instructions as you breathe.

1 Settle into your chosen position and just let breath come and go, in and out through the nose.

2 Notice when breath comes in and when it goes out. Just observe this coming and going.

3 Allow for breath to move at a natural pace. If there are quicker or slower breaths, notice them.

4 Then, begin to notice the rhythm of shifts from in-breath to out-breath. Inhalation/exhalation is a two-part rhythm: coming in, and going out; a circle of breath: one half going out, and one half coming in.

5 Then begin to notice the places where exhalation turns into inhalation. Watch these points, and acknowledge the turning of breath at them. Feel that breath rhythm is set by these places, these tiny pauses between inhalation and exhalation, and between exhalation and inhalation.

6 As your sense of breath rhythm becomes more acute, begin to notice how these pauses are not really pauses, but places of their own.

7 The rhythm of breath as you watch may now seem to shift from a rhythm based on the relationship between two: inhale and exhale; to a rhythm based on the relationship between four: inhale, and the place between inhale and exhale; exhale, and the place between it and the next inhale.

8 The circle of breath expands into this awareness, moving freely, effortlessly. Know that within this continuous rhythmic cycle of circles, everything is the same, and everything is changing. Breath keeps coming, and keeps changing.

9 Every breath is a complete rhythmic cycle – in, and pause, out, and pause. Each cycle leads away from the previous breath, and towards the coming breath.

10 Every rhythmic breath cycle contains within its circle all that we need to know. Things always change: the inhalation turns into the pause that follows; and the pause turns into the out-breath; and the out-breath turns into the pause that follows.

11 The individual breath cycle is complete, but its rhythm continues. Watch the rhythm continuing, containing within it the individual breath circles, cycles that lead one to the next.

12 Know that the truth of the breath circle is just this: right now, I am breathing in; right now I am watching the breath turn to leave; right now I am breathing out; right now I am waiting for the breath to turn back in.

13 Watching the rhythmic breath cycle, observe patterns of change, pause and release.

14 Each cycle of breath invites understanding that moments of change, or pause, or release, are always happening, over and over again – each rhythmic breath cycle is unique, and each one part of a pattern of change, pause and release.

Tips

Watch the breath closely enough to become respectful of its rhythm. If you are comfortable with the pauses at the end of exhale and inhale, then rest there momentarily without disrupting the natural rhythmic flow of the breath cycle. It is important not to extend this pause into enforced retention of breath. There should be no holding, just resting with the pause and waiting for the breath's rhythm to take you over into the next change. Noticing the turning moments between inhalation and exhalation can impart a sense of spaciousness. These pauses offer potential for profound insights and deep calm.

Once the Circle of breath becomes familiar, you can change the focus to respond to your present circumstances. For example, when life presents rapid change, it can be helpful to focus upon the stabilizing properties of the continuous circling of breath, reminding you that some things are always the same. This awareness can help you to cope with changes, especially those beyond your control, like how big your pregnant belly grows, or how many times your baby wakes each night. In times of uncertainty, reassurance that the 'breath is always the same' can be a helpful focus. On the other hand, in a situation where you feel stuck, it may be more encouraging to focus instead upon the process of change which the Circle of breath can reveal: the sense that it is always shifting, even within its constancy.

Full yogic breath – breath of life

Audio CD track 1

Based upon the previous practice's natural rhythm, Full yogic breath is the basis of all yoga breathing. It has three sections: abdominal breath, chest breath, and up to the collarbones. Instructions for individual parts are introduced cumulatively, building into a complete breathing pattern.

Paradoxically this is not really a 'technique' at all, since when you relax, inhaling and exhaling effectively, this is how the breath moves naturally. It is how you were born breathing; a full rhythm of complete breath that many adults forget as stress and tension conspire to restrict natural breathing patterns. If your breath is inadequate, you can feel low in energy simply because you are not getting enough oxygen, or are insufficiently clearing carbon dioxide.

Learning full yogic breathing reminds your body how to breathe effectively. It brings conscious awareness back to a process that can be so deeply unconscious that you may not even be aware of how inadequate to your needs your breath pattern is. The aim of bringing conscious awareness to the breath is not to maintain rigid control over its rhythms, but rather to allow for conscious expansion and improvement of breath capacity to become so familiar that it ultimately becomes second nature.

Full yogic breath part one: abdominal breath

This breath usually comes in and out through the nose. If that's not possible or comfortable for you, then allow breath to follow its easiest pathway.

1 Bring attention down to lowest part of abdomen.
2 Let breath create movement down between your navel and pubic bone.
3 Inhaling, allow your belly to expand.
4 Exhaling, feel your belly sink back towards your spine.

Tips

As the baby grows bigger, discernible movement of abdominal breath reduces. In the early weeks you may be able to feel as if the belly expands on inhalation and contracts on exhalation, but by the end of pregnancy, when the diaphragm is almost completely immobilized, this movement is barely detectable. At this time it can be helpful to establish an alternative connection with abdominal breath through the hands. Place the palms on lowest part of your belly, fingers pointing downward, and you may pick up a subtle gentle movement. If not, then simply direct the focus of awareness, through the palms' warmth, to that part of the belly. Send the nourishing energy of the breath down to that area by the shifting of your attention rather than by physical movement.

Abdominal breathing is calming and centring. During pregnancy it is a beautiful way to focus on the baby, 'breathing for two': imagining the extra space your baby gains on the inhalation, and consciously allowing the exhalation to release the baby deeper inside the warmth and safety of your body.

Full yogic breath part two: abdominal and chest breath together

This combines the previous practice with an expansion of breath higher into the chest. Especially in late pregnancy, after the movement of the diaphragm has reduced, chest breath is a very valuable practice, boosting energy and vitality.

Once you have established either a comfortable rhythm of abdominal movement, or a sense of energy travelling into the lower part of your belly through the palms, then you are ready to move breath higher up the body.

1 Allow chest to expand sideways, as breath moves in and up.
2 Feel each rib moving away from its neighbours, creating a sense of huge expansion in all directions, but especially from side to side.
3 Allow for this sideways movement to free space right up under armpits, as you continue to feel each rib moving up and out to create a big, welcoming space for incoming breath.
4 Allow upper back to expand, opening space between shoulder blades as breath moves up.
5 At the very end of the sideways rib movement, sense an upwards lift, carrying your breastbone higher and allowing for inhalation to lengthen further.
6 On exhalation allow whole chest to deflate.

Tips

The movement of expansion across the chest is much bigger than that in the belly. The sensation should be that the whole chest is opening sideways, to expand lung capacity. If you are lying on your back, feel the space between the shoulder blades opening up as they slide outwards and down against the floor. If you are sitting, rest the heels of your hands on the sides of your ribs, fingers pointing forwards, so that you can breathe into the hands and feel sideways expansion as your ribcage opens up.

Breathing fully from belly up into your chest is energizing and revitalizing. It raises the spirits and can encourage a more open-hearted, uplifted posture. This creates a welcome sense of space as the baby grows larger. It can help ease the feeling of panic that comes with breathlessness, and it is a powerful breath to build strength, courage and energy in the early stages of labour.

Full yogic breath part three: complete breath

Once the rhythm flows easily from belly up to chest and down again, proceed to the complete breath. This combines all three sections, abdominal, chest and up to the base of the throat to form the Full yogic breath. In this practice, the breath becomes like a wave flowing up the body on the inhalation and down the body on the exhalation.

1 Inhaling, feel breath rising all the way from pubic bone up to the top of the lungs at the base of throat.
2 Experience movement (physical or energetic) of your abdomen and full sideways expansion of ribs as breath fills lungs.
3 Maximize that expansion, taking ribs broader and wider as you fill lungs, feeling shoulder blades moving down and pressing forward, to allow for full inhalation.
4 Allow for lungs to expand completely, taking breath high, and sneaking in an extra top-up breath under collarbones.
5 Exhaling, allow movement of 'deflation' to flow down from base of throat to pubic bone.
6 Feel ribs coming back closer together, ribcage settling back to its starting position, and belly moving back towards spine.

Tips

Because this breath expansion takes awareness right up to the collarbones, sometimes the shoulders lift up towards the ears at the height of inhalation. This tends to close the front chest and bring tension into the neck and shoulders. To avoid it, keep shoulder blades drawn down your back, and move them in towards your spine as you inhale. This gives the forward and upward movement of the upper chest that allows for breath to move right up to the collarbones without hunching.

Using full lung expansion right up to the collarbones can be empowering and strengthening. It accesses the full power of the inhalation, and creates a fully open feeling across the front of the chest. Especially during late pregnancy, when the immobilization of the diaphragm compromises other aspects of the complete breath, inhaling up to the top of the lungs can increase vitality and alleviate breathlessness.

Take it easy; you should be relaxed enough to breathe completely, but at a comfortable rhythm and pace. After a while it should feel absolutely effortless. This is the simplest and most useful breath to cultivate throughout pregnancy: it energizes and calms. It is also a reassuring direct connection with your baby because, very often, Full yogic breath, which provides optimum oxygen supplies to the placenta, will prompt the baby to move. When the wave of the breath flows up and down the body, each inhalation nourishes and strengthens you and your baby, whilst each exhalation releases you both deeper into a state of healing rest.

Ujjayi breath – the victorious, conqueror or psychic breath

Audio CD track 2

This is the soft audible breath which everyone does every night when deeply asleep. It is often likened to the sound of a baby's breath as they sleep. Ujjayi slows both inhalation and exhalation by breathing through a slightly narrowed glottis. Adopting Ujjayi plays a clever yogic trick on the body, signalling it to enter a deep state of rest. Continued and regular use of Ujjayi breath can reduce high blood pressure, probably due to the calming effects of the lengthened inhales and exhales.

1 Tune into an effortless rhythm of breathing in and out through the nose.
2 Let face be soft.
3 Shift focus of mental attention to deep inside throat. Continue to breathe through nostrils, but feel as though breath is now coming and going through throat.
4 Feel breath passing over base of throat, almost as if you had by-passed your nose, and were breathing directly through imaginary gills. Breath is still actually coming in and out through nose, even though it feels as if it is in throat.

5 Allow there to be gentle sound in base of throat, rather like the soft beginnings of a snore (but not so hard as to make a snoring sound), or the breath you make at night as you sleep. Let this sound be very gentle, so that although throat is slightly constricted, it is soft. Keep on with the easy rhythm of breath.

6 Let there be the same quality of sound on the way in as on the way out.

Tips

Ujjayi can be done very quietly, so that only you and the baby can hear it. It can also be done more loudly, so that its sound 'drowns' your thoughts, like the sound of the waves of a far distant ocean. It can be helpful to imagine, as you listen to the sound of this distant ocean in your throat, that the breath is taking you to the source of all peace, a place of profound quiet, where you can rest absolutely undisturbed.

Some people feel a tightening sensation in the throat when practising Ujjayi. If this happens, let go of it for a while, and breathe as normal through the nose until the tightness releases. Then try at first only to create the soft sound on the exhale, and do not bother with the sound on the inhale until you feel absolutely at ease with the exhale. The temptation when learning Ujjayi is to create the sound at the expense of the rhythmic cycle of the breath. The soft sound of Ujjayi, when done properly, should enhance and not compromise the easy pace of the rhythmic breath cycle.

Some beginners find that it is easier to get the feel of this breath by making sighing sounds, exhaling through the mouth with a breathy sigh from deep in the throat. Once the sound of the breathy sigh creates the feeling of air moving across the back of the throat, then close the lips and continue to make the sighing sounds, but this time exhale through the nose. The resulting soft sound is Ujjayi breath.

Use this breath at the times when you need to centre yourself, or if you feel anxious or scared. See Chapter 08 for specific applications during labour and childbirth.

Golden thread exhalation

Audio CD track 3

The most valuable tool to promote relaxed acceptance, this breath focuses upon exhalation to ease the body into deep rest. Less a 'technique' than a way of becoming more aware of the power of the natural breath, this is basically a conscious practice of breath patterns adopted instinctively by many women in first stage labour. With each exhalation, you can let go deeper into healing stillness. The Golden thread works well in any position, but be aware that if you practise lying down you are likely to fall asleep.

1 Tune into a gentle pattern of breathing that is effortless. If you find it easy to do Full yogic breath use that as your starting point.

2 Take an extra yawn, release jaw, throat and teeth.

3 Allow there to be a very small space between top teeth and bottom teeth, between top lip and bottom lip; just enough gap that you might imagine a piece of tissue paper held between the lips, such a small gap that it is practically invisible.

4 Breathe in through nose.

5 Breathe out between slightly parted lips. Feel a fine cool breeze passing out between lips.

6 Cheeks, lips and face are relaxed. There is no pursing the lips. They are soft.

7 Feel breath travelling in through nose, and out through mouth. Allow the breath to be so fine that it feels as if a fine golden thread is spinning out between the lips. It's a thin, golden thread, like embroidery yarn, smooth and silky, spinning out with every exhalation.

8 Allow each exhalation to lengthen, without forcing, but simply letting the out-breath increase in length, as the golden thread of breath spins out into the air in front of you.

9 With each inhalation allow for breath to go in through nose and feel the breeze of exhalation travelling between the lips, into the air in front of your closed eyes.

10 Let the end of the golden thread carry the mental attention farther and farther away with each exhalation.

Tips

The heart of this practice is softness. You are not pursing the lips, or making them tight as if to whistle. The lips are soft, and the breath passing between them is silent and gentle. The lengthening of the exhalation is achieved effortlessly: simply because the gap through which the breath passes is so tiny, it takes a long time for all the breath to get out. There is no sense of force; simply watch the breath lengthen, following it out into the space in front of you. It should feel entirely effortless, completely comfortable and soothing. If you are struggling to exhale because the gap is too small, then simply widen the gap.

Any exhalation is an antidote to pain and tension. The Golden thread's extended exhalation makes this antidote more powerful. The longer the exhalation, the more effective this breath is as a form of pain and anxiety management. While staying within the comfortable limits of your own easy pace of breath, the longer the exhalation, the farther out the mental attention travels, and the more the body can relax into a quiet, mind-free space of healing and ease. The longer the exhalation is, the greater the distance between mind and body. Allow the Golden thread of the breath to travel out as far as is comfortable for you, and let the body make a voyage back to its natural healing state of easeful rest. When the mental awareness is at the far end of the long exhale, then the body can rest.

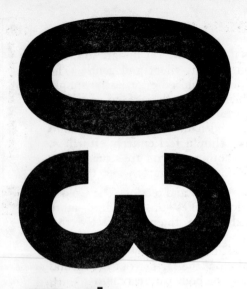

03 the physical body: earth

In this chapter you will learn:
- how to respond to the changing needs of the physical body during pregnancy
- how to do yoga poses that bring comfort, support mobility and build strength
- postures and sequences that can relieve minor ailments of pregnancy.

Earth gesture (prithvi mudra)

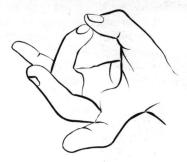

figure 3.1 Earth gesture

With hands resting palms up, comfortably on knees or thighs, lightly touch tip of ring finger to tip of thumb. The other fingers are relaxed. This hand gesture connects to the energy of the earth element, building qualities of support and solidity. It can be used together with core breaths (Chapter 02), or with postures (Chapters 03 and 04). It is also useful when you feel disconnected from the physical body, or need to be steadier or more grounded.

Getting grounded: being aware

The practice of physical postures in yoga is called *asana*, which is Sanskrit for 'seat'. Whilst the aim of asana is ultimately to perfect your ability to sit comfortably ready for meditation, there are many beneficial side effects to their practice. Appropriate asana practice can encourage a healthy range of motion in the body, counteracting stiffness, building strength and stability, increasing vitality and promoting efficient functioning of all bodily systems. Its primary benefit, however, is to increase awareness of the physical body. During pregnancy this increased awareness is helpful to develop an understanding and sensitive response to the many adaptations which your body makes to the presence of the growing baby within.

In this chapter, the asanas are grouped together in families of postures with a shared base. Each base position offers particular benefits: the transitional moves (p. 27) promote ease of motion between different positions; the resting postures (p. 33) enable you to find comfortable ways to encourage healing and restorative quiet; the cat family poses (p. 38) encourage stability, optimal foetal position, and provide relief for lower back, pelvis and groin strain; the cat base lunge poses (p. 44) create freedom of movement for the upper back and encourage easier breath; and the three point balances (p. 47) offer opportunities for graceful, energizing poses to boost vitality. Back on the ground, the seated poses (p. 52) promote a deep connection with the earth, which is both restful, stabilizing and energizing; whilst the poses in the pelvic movement family (p. 73) relieve stiffness and pain in the lower back, promoting an energizing freedom of movement from the body's core. The standing poses (p. 79) strengthen back and legs, creating space and ease of motion in the spine; the squatting family (p. 90) are all poses to build leg strength, boost pelvic circulation and enable you to discover your own comfortable open pelvis position for birth. The asanas in the wall supported family (p. 96) offer a unique combination of resting and strengthening options to improve posture and build strength in supported poses; whilst the dynamic warrior adaptations (p. 104) work from the ground up to encourage good posture, stamina and freedom of breath and energy. In all these poses, the process of 'getting grounded' has the positive implication of building a connection with the earth that boosts vitality and promotes clarity of understanding about how best to respond to the changing needs of the physical body in order to encourage the optimal functioning of its many systems.

In yoga, the element associated with the physical body is earth (prithvi), which has qualities of heaviness, nurturing and solidity, dampness and firmness. To be in harmony with the qualities of earth during pregnancy is to experience a contented acceptance of the growing weight and altering form of the body, and to perceive that these changes promote a secure connection with the earth, with all things that grow, ripen and need to be nurtured.

From a yoga perspective, the pregnant body is a physical manifestation of unconditional love: in physiological terms the needs of the growing baby always come first, and your bodily systems adapt to provide the environment and nourishment needed by your baby. This experience of unconditional love is the most refined form of the nurturing qualities of the earth element. But whilst other experiences of higher forms of love may be consciously chosen as part of a spiritual path, or from convictions of faith, the pregnant body does not request permission to make these changes; the nurturing qualities of earth simply take over the physical form of the pregnant mother.

She becomes heavier, rounder, slower, and every system of her body adapts its functioning to support the presence of the unborn baby. If you are attuned to the qualities of earth, these changes may be embraced happily, but to be out of harmony with the earth element in pregnancy can manifest as a sense of resentment or fear about the growing body or its changing shape, resistance to the slower, quieter pace which it demands, or discomfort with new ways of moving and being, which more readily accommodate the growth of the baby within.

With sensitive practice of appropriate yoga postures, ease and grace with increasing weight and other changes come through heightened awareness of the needs of the physical body. This encourages appreciation of the earth element, which results in a more joyous acceptance of 'groundedness' as a benefit, a source of stability, strength and nurturing. All of these qualities are essential to a positive experience of the transition to motherhood, or an expansion of mother love to accommodate the arrival of new siblings.

Adapting your yoga practice to bodily changes

Bodily changes and commonly experienced discomforts during pregnancy will impact on your yoga practice. Every system of your body is changed in some way by pregnancy, and the effects are noticeable from the very first weeks. Some of these changes are especially significant to women doing yoga postures, and it is important to be aware of the impact which they may have upon yoga practice in order to adjust techniques to meet your physical needs. In fact, many of these maternal adaptations to pregnancy are more easily accommodated through the practice of yoga.

Joints during pregnancy become more supple, often moving into a wider range of motion than you would normally experience. This increased range of motion is caused by the presence of hormones, especially relaxin, whose primary role is to soften joints and ligaments to allow 'give' in the pelvis and facilitate the birth of your baby. But whilst relaxin's 'target joints' are those in the pelvis, increased suppleness from softening ligaments and joints is experienced everywhere. This is an important consideration for pregnant yoga students. Whilst it can create freedom of movement, it can also be a source of discomfort, as joints lack the usual structures of support provided by normally inelastic ligaments.

Taking yoga postures into the additional range of motion offered by the soft ligaments of pregnancy can create strain and possibly cause permanent damage to joints, or uneven wear in later life. For this reason, it is wisest to contain the opportunity for stretch offered by yoga poses, and to keep the range of movement within normal range. Some people are naturally more flexible or stiffer than others, so the best way to ascertain your safe limits of motion during pregnancy is to refer to the range of motion achievable prior to pregnancy. This is a clearer reference point for women who have practised yoga before; they should simply continue to observe their usual base positions, especially in the seated wide-angled pose (p. 53), but if you have not practised yoga before pregnancy, the safest advice is to proceed with caution and always work with a sense of comfort and ease. Feeling a stretch in the middle portion of a muscle is usually an indication of well-directed effort, but feeling any pulling or 'give' in a joint, or at the places where muscles attach to joints (for example around the inner knee) is to be avoided. To maintain the structural integrity of the body, direct equal focus the building of stability and strength in a pose, and do not simply focus on the stretch it provides. Tips following the instructions for the poses explain how to keep this balance between strength and flexibility.

The suppleness of pregnant ligaments not only impacts upon safety in yoga postures, but also creates challenges and opportunities for maintaining comfortable posture in everyday activities such as standing, sitting and walking. Spinal curves alter during pregnancy, as a result of the increasing weight of the uterus, the hormonal effects on the joints, and the changing position and size of the baby. As the baby grows, the weight of the womb pulls on supporting ligaments and muscles of the spine, especially increasing the strain in the lower back, so that pain in this area, and indeed throughout the length of the spine, is very common (but often avoidable) during pregnancy. A sequence of postures to prevent and reduce back pain is on page 183.

Back pain in pregnancy can be exacerbated by changes to the structure of other joints, for example, increased joint suppleness in the feet can cause arches to spread and flatten. Because these arches are the foundation of good posture, their flattening can reduce the effectiveness of the support system for the spine, especially the lower back. Practices on page 183 describe how yoga may remedy and prevent this.

Throughout the instructions, you will also find pointers on managing pain or discomfort in the pelvic joints. Often referred to as 'pubic symphysis dysfunction' (PSD or SPD), pain in the front joint of the pelvis, at the pubic bone, has recently become more widely diagnosed, and manifests as sharp pain when walking or when carrying weight unevenly on either leg, for example, when standing on one leg, putting on trousers, or getting into and out of cars by stepping the foot wide, thus shifting weight onto one leg. This experience can range from mild discomfort to utterly debilitating constant pain. At the severe end of the spectrum, women may be referred to an obstetric physiotherapist (see p. 236). At the more manageable end of the spectrum, the enhanced postural awareness and muscle strength building of some yoga asanas can be effective in prevention and reduction of pain. Sequences to manage this experience are on page 184. Be aware also that certain yoga asanas are to be avoided because they may exacerbate the discomfort of PSD. The general rule is to avoid any poses that bring uneven weight through legs and feet. These practices are identified in the 'Cautions' section of the instructions.

Yoga offers a system of postural support and management that can help to prevent or minimize difficulties caused by musculoskeletal changes during pregnancy. On a more positive note, the combination of increased joint suppleness during pregnancy and heightened awareness of postural change which yoga promotes can also bring about profound healing and postural improvements that last a lifetime.

Case study – Charlotte

I attended yoga classes during my first pregnancy and was delighted to discover that the constant back pain, which I had experienced since adolescence as a result of a riding accident, had begun to reduce during pregnancy. For me, the hormonal effects of joint softening had created ease of movement and freedom from pain. Yoga poses enhanced this effect by improving my posture so much that by the end of the pregnancy I was virtually pain free. When I returned two years later pregnant with my second child, the improvements had lessened slightly post-natally, but the postural awareness I had learnt during my first pregnancy assisted in the management of the back pain ever since. On my second pregnancy, the improvements continued, and I have never since experienced the degree of pain I had prior to the first pregnancy.

In this case, and many others, the changes of pregnancy, supported by yoga, provides a great opportunity for healing and improved well-being that extends far beyond the nine months of gestation.

The other major physical adaptations to pregnancy which impact directly upon yoga practice are water retention around joints resulting in swelling (most frequently around ankles), and increases to heart rate and blood volume. In the first case, it can be uncomfortable to put weight on swollen joints, for example by kneeling back directly on heels. Any poses that might aggravate the discomfort of swollen and tender joints have additional instructions for the use of props to protect affected joints.

In the second case, there a number of issues related to changes in the cardiovascular system during pregnancy which all point to the wisdom of keeping yoga practice in pregnancy very slow. This is because blood volume increases by nearly half, so the heart is pumping much harder and faster than usual, even during a resting state. As well as causing breathlessness (discussed in more detail in the next chapter), this also means that pregnant women are usually warmer than usual, and moving too fast can cause overheating. Blood pressure also tends to lower during pregnancy, and this can increase the likelihood of fainting. So to minimize breathlessness, overheating and/or fainting, it is best to keep yoga practices slow and steady during pregnancy. Rapid or over-vigorous physical exercise in later pregnancy will redirect blood to the muscles and away from the placenta that provides the baby's blood supply. This is not advisable.

For some women, changes to the circulation during pregnancy, combined with the effects of hormones which dilate the blood vessels, can cause increased pressure in leg and pelvic veins, leading to varicose veins and haemorrhoids. To avoid exacerbating these possible difficulties during yoga practice, tips are given about comfortable sitting options.

Some women also experience other adaptations to pregnancy that can sometimes cause discomfort, such as nausea, constipation, heartburn and carpal tunnel syndrome. Although these have a less direct impact upon yoga practice, it is important to avoid poses that can exacerbate the discomfort they may cause. Guidance about this is given in the 'Tips' section of the instructions.

During pregnancy, you need to 'breathe for two' to meet the oxygen needs of the growing baby. There are also changes to the functioning of the respiratory system, which are addressed in more detail in the next chapter, and changes to the nervous system, which are described in Chapters 04 and 05.

Yoga postures (asanas)

Following the instructions and diagrams are suggested tips, modifications and cautions for safe and comfortable practice at each stage of pregnancy. Please read all the way through the advice for a particular pose before starting to do it.

Each family of postures is grouped around a base pose. This makes them easier to learn, and also helps you to create flowing sequences. The posture families are organized with the most accessible poses first, and are preceded by a set of transitional moves enabling you to come into all base positions with ease, and to move between postures with grace and comfort. The supported restorative poses in the seated group give the essential benefits of base positions without the need for physical effort.

Transitional moves

Yoga asanas are a repertoire of movement and posture to promote strength, flexibility, stability, grace and heightened awareness. The process of entering and leaving the final posture is always as important as the asana itself. In pregnancy, when you are coping with many different bodily changes that alter your size and sense of balance, it is especially important to be aware of the transitional moves leading into and out of poses. Use the simple movement and awareness pointers below to get comfortably into and out of the poses that follow. The transitional moves teach you to learn how to move your body safely, with grace and control. Learning to move with yoga awareness helps you to adapt everyday movement patterns to the needs of the changing pregnant body.

Standing to all fours

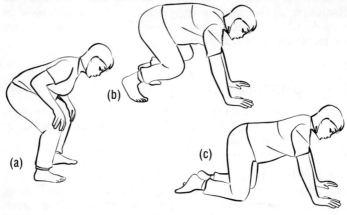

figure 3.2a, b, c Standing to all fours

- Feet slightly wider than hips, either parallel, or turned out to a maximum of 'five to one', knees bent slightly.
- Bend knees deeper, lowering towards floor.
- Reach hands and arms forward, and down to floor.
- Spread fingers wide and take weight in hands, shoulder width apart.
- Keeping knees wide, lower them to the floor simultaneously, so both knees touch ground at same time.

Tips

If it seems too far to reach down to the floor, put your hands on the top of a chair, and then walk them down to the chair seat before coming to the ground. As you gain confidence, take hands to chair seat first, and then down to the floor. Gradually reduce height until you can shift onto a low table or settee seat to ease down to the floor. Make sure chair is stable before giving it your whole weight.

Cautions

If you experience pain in the pubic joint, be especially sure to bring both knees down to the ground at precisely the same moment to avoid transferring weight unevenly into the pelvis.

All fours to sitting and back up

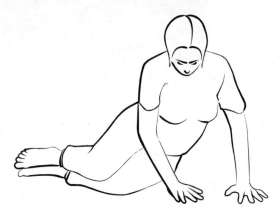

figure 3.3 All fours to sitting

- Knees hip width apart. Toes tucked under, or pointed back.
- Spread fingers wide and position hands at shoulder width, slightly ahead of shoulders.
- Slowly walk hands around to one side, keeping a space between hands and body.
- When hands reach as far round as they will comfortably go, then lower hips to floor, being careful to let knees slide slightly and gently open.
- Readjust knees and feet to your chosen sitting position.

Tips

If you experience any pain or instability in the pelvis, either in the pubic symphysis or in the sacroiliac joints, then keep knees closer together from the start, squeezing inner thighs and engaging buttocks to limit degree of movement in pelvic joints as you shift position. Be particularly attentive to taking weight firmly in hands and through arms, to keep knees close together as you lower hips. This minimizes strain on pelvis.

To move back from sitting to all fours, reverse direction of the preceding instructions, using upper body strength to raise pelvis to all fours position.

All fours to floor

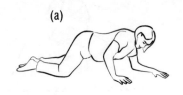

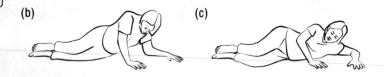

figure 3.4 a, b, c All fours to floor

- Hands shoulder width apart, knees hip width apart.
- Walk hands further away from you. To lie on left side, move left hand ahead, beyond shoulder level. Keep right hand close to body at shoulder level.
- As hands move into position, keep fingers spread wide and use upper body strength to lower hips to floor.
- Keep most of weight coming down into right hand until left side of body is in contact with floor.
- Support lying pose as needed (p. 34).

Tips

If you have pain in the pelvis, keep knees squeezed more closely together as you shift position.

Lying to sitting

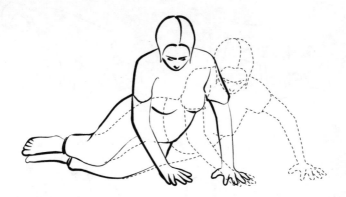

figure 3.5 Lying to sitting

- If you are lying on your back, roll over to side.
- From side lying, bring both hands to floor in front of you at chest height, shoulder width apart, elbows bent.
- Spread fingers wide and take weight of upper body through arms and hands down into floor.
- Bend knees and gently spiral body over towards hands, using upper body strength (not abdominal effort) to support shift in position.
- Bend elbows more to enable you to bring knees down to floor.
- Shift into all fours position, straightening elbows.
- From all fours, follow instructions (p. 29) to transfer into your chosen sitting posture.

Tips

To minimize pain in the pelvis, keep knees together as they roll to the floor.

All fours to standing

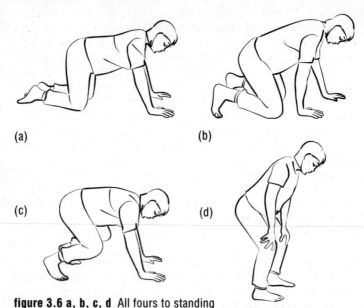

(a)

(b)

(c)

(d)

figure 3.6 a, b, c, d All fours to standing

- Knees and feet hip width apart, wider if that feels comfortable.
- Take weight on hands and spread fingers wide.
- Walk hands back towards knees.
- As hands come closer to knees use arm strength to lift both knees up from floor simultaneously and take weight into toes and balls of feet.
- Straighten arms and shift weight back across the outer edges of soles of feet into heels.
- Keep knees bent as you raise hands from floor.
- Rest palms on knees and walk hands up thighs until standing.

Tips

The wider apart the feet and knees are to begin with, the easier this transition is. Keep toes pointing forwards as much as possible, and not turned out to side. If it feels like a long way up, then practise near a chair or sofa, using the seat as a staging post for hands between floor and standing. If you experience pain in the pelvis, be extra sure to lift both knees up from the floor simultaneously.

Case study – Rose

Rose was 15 weeks pregnant with her second baby when she developed severe pain in the front of her pelvis. She was having difficulty walking, rolling over in bed, and lifting and carrying her two-year-old daughter. She was diagnosed with pubic symphysis dysfunction (PSD), and in order to minimize the pain, Rose began to pay special attention to transitional movements in the pregnancy yoga classes she was attending. She focused on keeping the legs closer, taking weight through the arms, adjusting her standing and walking posture and using her pelvic floor muscles for additional support. She transferred this postural awareness into her daily activities and within a week she was able to push her daughter in the buggy without pain. She also obtained a referral to an obstetric physiotherapist, who prescribed exercises to support the pelvic joints in ways very similar to the yoga work she was already doing. Rose maintained her pain-free state for the remainder of her pregnancy by continuing to observe the postural awareness that had helped to reduce the pain. She said: 'Yoga and the advice I received from my teacher helped to eradicate the PSD. The classes made me much more aware of my movements and I stopped doing things that put pressure on my pubic symphysis, so after my fifth month of pregnancy I didn't have any pain at all'.

Resting postures: lying comfortably

Many pregnant women find it a challenge to discover comfortable and sustainable resting positions. These resting postures use props and supports to assist the pregnant body to relax completely, maximizing its capacity to heal, grow and repair. Once the skills of self-propping are learnt, you can make yourself very peaceful in these poses. They can be used during yoga sessions for deep relaxation (Chapters 05 and 06), or at night to get comfortable in bed. The instructions below describe the basic props necessary to support the poses. If you are intending to rest longer than five minutes then cover yourself with a blanket and cover your eyes with an eyebag or scarf. A deeper state of rest is achieved when the body is warm and the eyes are in darkness.

Of all the many poses taught in pregnancy yoga classes, these are without doubt the ones that women most relish. You will find additional restorative poses in different base positions on pages 36, 40, 60, 69, 71 and 72.

Lateral lying with support (modified matsya kridasana)

This is the best restorative pose for all stages of pregnancy. It can be done without props, for short periods, but for any longer than a couple of minutes, appropriate supports make it much more comfortable.

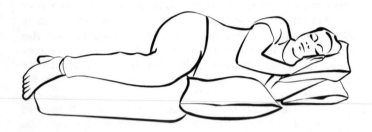

figure 3.7 Lateral lying with support

You will need: a pillow or two for your head, and also perhaps one to put under your bump, and either a bolster or stack of yoga blocks (six is optimal) to support top leg.

Ensure leg support is high, firm and long enough to support the entire lower leg (from above knee right down to ankle) at hip height. This means leg support should be at least as high as your hips are wide. Check this by placing a hand on either hip and then comparing distance between your two hands with height of prop. They should be about the same. If the prop is very much smaller than this distance, your top leg will drag down, pulling from the sacrum. This may (especially if you are in the pose for a long while) cause discomfort in the lower back. If height of prop matches width of pelvis, then the upper leg is supported effortlessly level with hips.

- Use transitional movements (p. 27) to lower gently down into a side-lying position.
- Have underneath leg either straight, or slightly bent.

- Bend top leg and support it so that whole length of lower leg, from just above knee to foot, is resting on top surface of support.
- Once legs are comfortable, place pillow under belly to support weight of bump, and adjust arms and head.
- Place underneath arm in whichever of the following three positions feels most comfortable:
  - out in front, resting on floor at shoulder level,
  - stretched up above head, underneath supporting pillows,
  - or extended slightly behind body, so that there is a slight roll in front of body.
- If underneath hand is out in front, or back behind, then position pillows one under shoulder and one between ear and shoulder to support neck. If hand is above head, place arm under pillows.
- Slide shoulders down away from ears and gently tuck in chin.
- Allow body to settle into supports.
- Establish an easy rhythm of breath.

Tips

Many pregnant women worry about which side to lie on. Some midwives and pregnancy yoga teachers argue that in late pregnancy, lying on the left side increases the likelihood that baby will come into an optimal position for birth (p. 195), and others say it does not matter. Many yoga teachers and midwives also point out that the blood vessels leading to and from the uterus get a better supply of oxygenated blood to the baby if the mother lies on her left. In terms of ensuring optimal blood supply to the baby, then left side lying is certainly better than supine (on your back).

Obviously at night, when shifting positions in sleep, you often end up on your back. This is a perfectly natural part of movement patterns in sleep and is nothing to worry about. It is not possible to stick resolutely to side lying every minute you are asleep, but when in a situation (like a yoga session) where it is possible to make a conscious choice, then it seems wisest to opt for side lying. Many women instinctively turn to rest on the left, but if that is not comfortable for you, then lie on the right. The most important thing is to enjoy the posture you have chosen.

Semi-supine and modified corpse pose (savasana)

Cautions

These two back-lying poses are not advisable after 25–30 weeks of pregnancy (or sooner, if carrying twins), when the increasing weight of baby and placenta can compress blood vessels which supply oxygen to the baby. After this time, or whenever lying on the back doesn't feel comfortable, then use side lying instead.

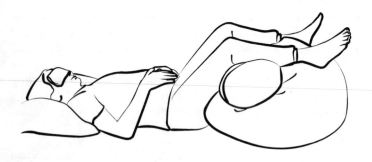

figure 3.8 Semi-supine with support

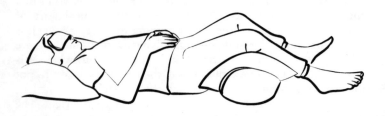

figure 3.9 Corpse with support (hands in your mudra)

The 'corpse' is the classic yoga relaxation pose, in which the physical body lies flat out on the back, dead still. During pregnancy, changes to the lower back curve make it wiser and more comfortable to bend knees to reduce strain in lumbar spine. The most comfortable way to do this is with support under knees. These two options provide different levels of support, and most pregnant women find that once their bump begins to swell, they prefer the higher level of support.

You will need: a pillow or two for your head and either a chair (the seat of a sofa works well), or a beanbag and/or bolster to support lower legs.

- Use transitional movements (p. 27) to lower gently down into side lying (p. 34).
- Use arm strength to roll over onto your back, keeping knees bent.
- For lower level of support, simply place prop under knees to create a comfortable bend. The height of support directly impacts on lumbar (lower back) curve, so experiment to find what suits.
- When bend in knees feels right, place pillow under head.
- For higher level of support, position prop so you can bend knees and lift feet and lower legs to rest calves on support. Ensure backs of knees are in contact with front edge of support.
- Either place feet close together and allow knees to drop to either side or keep feet hip width apart and shins parallel.
- For both levels of support, slide tops of shoulders down away from ears and either have hands resting by sides, palms up, a little away from body or bring palms to rest on belly. Yoni mudra is often comfortable in this pose.

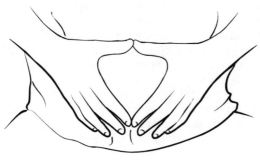

figure 3.10 Hands in yoni mudra

- If your elbows do not touch the ground, then place cushions beneath them.

Tips

If you experience pelvic pain, keep legs squeezed together as you roll on to your back. Be sure higher prop is at a level that supports back of knees. If it feels too low, raise top edge of prop by adding a rolled blanket under knees.

Case study – Emma

Emma was 30 weeks pregnant with her first baby when she began to find it impossible to sleep at night. She especially valued the restorative sections of the pregnancy yoga classes: 'This is always my favourite part of the session because I get to sleep'. One week she turned up to class reporting ten consecutive nights of not being able to sleep at all. She was exhausted. During that session, she paid particular attention to her alignment and support in side lying, and discovered that she needed more pillows and a higher level of leg support than she had been using at home. She enjoyed the 20-minute relaxation during the class and returned the following week to tell us: 'Learning the yoga propping helped me to get more comfortable in bed at night so that I could sleep'.

Cat family (all fours)

Encouraging stability, optimal foetal position, and providing relief for lower back, pelvis and groin strain.

This all fours base position is a stable and comfortable starting point for many postures, and provides helpful transitions between other poses. Essentially, the all fours poses allow for the growing baby to hang in the hammock of your belly, freeing your pelvis and the lower back from strain caused by downward pressure and weight of the uterus. This can be a great comfort and relief throughout all stages of pregnancy. The positive experiences described by Lucy whilst pregnant with her first baby are very typical: 'I loved these cat poses most of all. The figure of eight move was particularly relaxing and felt like it was doing good for me and my baby. It just loosened everything up and really helped me to relax.'

Cautions

In all Cat variations, ensure that the lower back curve does not dip further than in a normal standing posture. The classic yoga practice of this pose places a deep inward curve in the lumbar spine on inhale, but this is not advisable during pregnancy, when the lordosis (inward curve) of the lower back naturally deepens to accommodate the growing bump, making the lower back vulnerable. If this lordosis is allowed to deepen during all fours poses in pregnancy, it can exacerbate the tendency to lower back pain.

All Cat poses are best done on a mat that provides sufficient soft support for the knees. If being on all fours causes knee discomfort, then use a cushion or folded blanket for extra padding. If your wrists are uncomfortable with palms flat on floor, then either place a rolled blanket under heel of hand to change angle of wrist bend; or make fists and rest on top of fists instead of palms; or else take no weight through hands at all by propping entire length of forearm from elbow to wrist on a flat support at elbow height, for example by resting forearms on a low table or stack of yoga blocks. You can rest forearms flat on floor to alleviate wrist strain, but this tips head lower, limiting upper back movements and sometimes aggravating nausea or heartburn, so it is better to support forearms at a higher level. If wrist problems persist, see p. 187 for remedies and pain management.

Cat (majariasana)

With its full stretch, and rhythmic movement in time with the breath, this practice optimizes mobility along length of spine.

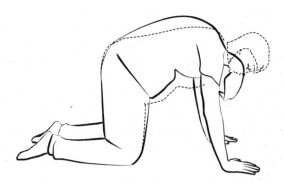

figure 3.11 Cat

- Transition down all fours (p. 28).
- Use knee or wrist supports necessary for comfort.
- Knees about hip width apart, hands shoulder width apart slightly ahead of shoulders with fingers spread wide and strong.
- Breathe fully, either in and out through nose, or with Golden thread exhalation (p. 18). Let rhythm of breath determine pace of movements.
- Inhaling, with back as flat as possible, move shoulders down away from ears, allowing chest to expand and move forwards a little.
- Exhaling, tuck chin into throat, tuck tailbone in and down, and round entire length of spine, creating plenty of space especially between shoulder blades.
- Follow natural rhythm of breath and alternate between these two positions: flat back on inhale, and round back on exhale.
- Feel that rhythm of breath is creating physical movements.
- Repeat five rounds, and as familiarity and comfort grow, increase repetitions to ten.
- Rest in Hare pose (instructions below), with supports if needed.

Hare pose rest (shashankasana)

This is the ideal resting posture to follow all Cat based poses.

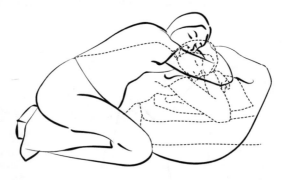

figure 3.12 Hare pose rest (with high support)

- From Cat, move knees a little wider apart, with enough space to take your belly forward and down between knees easily. If it feels more comfortable, let toes move close together as knees move wider apart.
- Exhaling, round spine.
- Move buttocks back towards heels, keeping hands in place.
- Rest buttocks on heels and allow forehead to rest on support. If comfortable, remain here for up to ten breaths, or as long as feels good. If there is any discomfort, then come out and adjust as described below.

Tips

Whilst Hare pose is calming and restful for many pregnant women in early pregnancy, many women prefer higher support as the bump grows. A stack of blocks (two or three) or cushions between the feet provides a higher resting place for buttocks. A cushion, bolster or folded blanket gives a higher resting place for the head. Adjust height until it feels right: instead of being horizontal, the body rests on a slight forward incline, using a chair, bean bag, or even the seat or the back of a sofa. This higher support is very necessary if the standard pose tends to induce nausea, and/or aggravate heartburn or breathlessness. If knees or ankles feel uncomfortable when buttocks drop back, then place cushions or a blanket behind knees before moving buttocks down.

Flowing Hare-to-Cat swoop (shashank-bhujangasana)

This is a flowing rhythmic alternation between the two previous poses, running them together into one smooth movement in time with the breath.

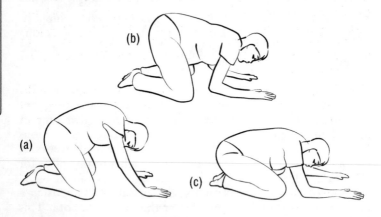

figure 3.13 a, b, c Flowing Hare-to-Cat swoop

- Begin in Cat with black flat (p. 39).
- Move knees a little wider apart, with enough space to take your belly forward between them easily. If it feels more comfortable, let toes move closer as knees move wider.
- Breath fully. Let rhythm of breath determine pace of movements.
- Exhaling, round back.
- Keeping spine rounded, maintain firm connection between hands and mat as you continue to exhale and lower buttocks towards heels.
- At end of exhale, sense you have moved as far back towards heels as is comfortable (Hare pose).
- Inhaling, bend elbows and move forwards, keeping as low to mat as you can.
- When you reach thumbs, straighten elbows, lifting body back into flat-back position.
- Exhaling, round spine and drop back towards buttocks.
- Continue for a couple of rounds, exhaling with rounded spine as you move back to heels, and inhaling with a flat back as you move forward to hands.

- After three repetitions, pause, evaluate your response and either rest, or repeat up to ten rounds.
- Rest in Hare pose, supported as needed (p. 40).

Tips

As elbows bend to support forward motion of body, there are two directions in which they can move. Letting elbows stick out sideways gives more freedom of movement but less strength; tucking elbows into sides of body challenges range of movement but builds strength. Choose whichever option seems most appropriate, or alternate between the two.

If dropping buttocks back to heels feels awkward, and you do not get very far, it can be more comfortable to have a support to sit on as for Hare pose, so place a stack of blocks (two or three) or cushions between feet.

Circles and figures of eight

These rhythmic movements optimize mobility, relieve stiffness and have a calming, hypnotic effect. They also create soothing rocking movement for the unborn child.

- Breathe fully in Cat (p. 39), with padding as needed.
- Keeping a flat back, let rhythm of breath continue easily throughout movements.
- Imagine central point of a circle between knees, and slowly circle hips clockwise around this point, letting size of circle increase or decrease as feels comfortable.
- After about ten rounds, change direction and repeat.
- Pause, shift movement up body so that imaginary central point of circle is now between hands.
- Circle shoulders and upper body clockwise, and then anticlockwise, moving freely and easily.
- Connect shoulder circles with hip circles, as if drawing a figure of eight by moving hips in one direction and shoulders in the other.
- Feel central cross-over point in figure of eight, and savour moments when lower circles cross into upper and vice versa.
- When you have moved enough in one direction, change direction and repeat.
- At end of sequence do one round of Cat.
- Rest in Hare pose, supported as needed (p. 40).

Cat base lunge family

Creating freedom of movement for the upper back and encouraging easier breath.

These poses provide a stable base for energizing and mobilizing movement options throughout pregnancy. They also make excellent birthing positions (p. 204).

Cautions

This position shifts weight into one knee, causing an uneven load on the pelvis. Proceed with caution if you experience pelvic pain, and if pose is uncomfortable, do not step foot forward, but use 'high kneeling' with both knees on floor and buttocks raised.

Cat lunge

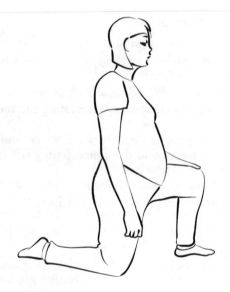

figure 3.14 Cat lunge

- From Cat step left foot forward to outside of left hand.
- Inhaling, raise torso, resting left elbow on left knee.
- Exhaling, settle base position, adjusting feet if necessary.

Cat lunge with arm circles

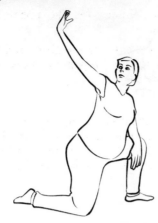

figure 3.15 Cat lunge with arm circles

- From Cat lunge, circle left arm, reaching up and back on inhale and down on exhale.
- Repeat up to ten rounds and change direction.
- Return to Cat, switch leg positions for lunge and repeat on other side.
- Rest in Hare pose (p. 40).

Tips

Even if you do not usually use knee support in Cat, this pose takes more weight through the knee, and it is wise to have padding, especially if you do a number of repetitions. Circling with elbow straight builds arm strength, and circling with elbow bent uses deep core muscles that support the torso: try both. This pose works well in a simple sequence with Cat, and in Sun and Moon flows (p. 177–9).

Half squat circles

These rhythmic movements are easier to sustain than a full squat and can help you discover the most open position for your pelvis.

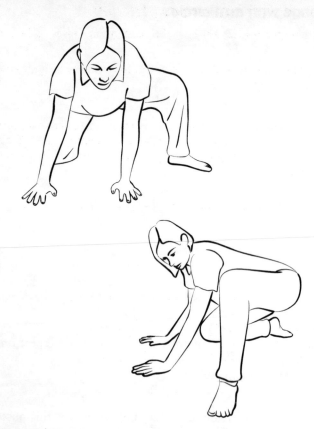

figure 3.16 Half squat circles (front and side)

- From Cat step left foot forward to outside of left hand.
- Adjust position of right foot until pelvic floor feels comfortably open.
- Inhale, fingers wide, shifting weight forward and circling left.
- Exhale, sink weight backwards and circle right.
- Circle in time with breath for three rounds, then change direction.
- Return to Cat and repeat on other side.

Tips

Ensure whole foot remains in contact with floor as you circle. If you find that your heel raises as you circle, it may be that foot is too far out, so bring it closer in, and/or further back.

Three point balancing family

Offering opportunities for graceful, energizing poses to boost vitality.

These options use the stable base of Cat to open into elegant and spacious balances.

Cautions

Because weight is shifted mainly to one leg, these balances are not suitable if you have pubis symphysis dysfunction. If so, keep knees in Cat and only change arm position for Half moon variation (p. 50).

Tiger preparation (vyaghrasana)

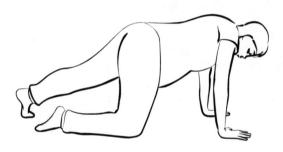

figure 3.17 Tiger preparation

- Breathe fully in Cat.
- Keep hands strong, fingers spread wide.
- Raise left knee from floor, keeping toes and ball of left foot pressing into floor as leg straightens.
- Exhaling, lengthen leg away into heel of left foot, extending from hip to foot along back of leg.
- Inhaling, squeeze buttocks to hold leg straight and strong.
- After three or five rounds, lower left knee and repeat on right.

Tiger variation part one

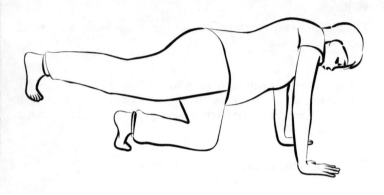

figure 3.18 Tiger variation part one

- Follow instructions for Tiger preparation, but instead of keeping foot on floor, raise extended leg to buttock level.
- Inhaling, use buttock strength and leg muscles to hold extended leg steady, foot flexed.
- Exhaling, lower straight leg to floor and bend knee.
- Repeat twice more on right and then switch to left.
- If you can hold leg steady for one round of breath, repeat, alternating flexed foot with pointed foot.

Tips

Keep hips level and steady by engaging buttock muscles, and do not raise leg higher than hips. If you feel wobbly, check hand position and adopt a wider Cat base. Keeping a steady gaze helps maintain balance.

Tiger variation part two

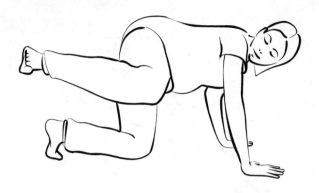

figure 3.19 Tiger variation part two

Only if you feel strong and steady with Tiger part one, this option provides further opportunities to mobilize and strengthen hips and legs. The same cautions apply as for Tiger.

- Follow instructions for Tiger until right leg is lifted and extended behind.
- Inhaling, hold right leg steady and turn foot so toes point to right side.
- Exhaling, bend right knee and draw it towards right side of body, keeping knee and foot lifted at buttock level.
- Inhaling, extend leg straight behind and bring foot back to floor.
- Do two more rounds on right before switching to left.

Tips

Use strength of back and buttocks to stabilize balance. As you bend knee towards you, turn head to check on its position. This can help to maintain knee at buttock level. Flexing foot also helps to hold knee level.

Half moon variation (ardha chandrasana)

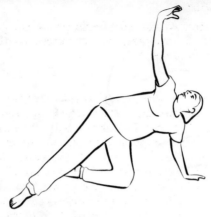

figure 3.20 Half moon variation

An elegant easy balance that opens the chest, lifts the spirits and promotes vitality throughout pregnancy.

- Follow instructions for Tiger preparation.
- Once right knee is straight, keep foot on floor, but turn ankle to bring inner edge of foot to rest on floor with toes pointing right, foot flexed.
- Slide foot further right to widen distance between left knee and right foot.
- Inhaling, reach right arm forwards, brushing ear with upper arm as it moves in front of head and then straight up above in an arc.
- Exhaling, reach arm back towards feet and down to floor.
- Repeat arm circle, reaching forward and upward on each inhale, and drawing backward and downward on each exhale.
- Repeat up to ten rounds on right before switching to left.
- To increase focusing and balancing effects of this practice, place hands in Earth gesture (p. 21) as they circle.

Tips

To begin with, keep head and neck steady as you get used to arm action. As motion becomes familiar, turn head to watch movements.

Cat–Dog–Cat variation (Majariasana to adho mukha svanasana)

This pair of postures work well together, with the grounded stability of the Cat providing gentle access to the more challenging inversion of the Dog.

Cautions

During pregnancy take the transition into Dog very slowly indeed, gauging your response to the inversion and returning to Cat if you feel any discomfort, dizziness, sickness or rapid change in body temperature. Some women, even those who have great familiarity with Dog, discover to their surprise that it can be a very unpleasant pose to practise in pregnancy. This can be due to a number of factors, including the position of the baby and/or the placenta, changes in blood pressure, or digestive disturbances such as heartburn or nausea. These factors can alter from day to day, so always check your present response to the pose even if it has been comfortable in the past.

Dog pose is an inversion, with heart raised higher than head. This places some challenging demands on the pregnant body, and it is sensible to treat the pose with caution. That said, some women find it to be a source of great delight and vitality, and enjoy taking the weight of the bump away from the pelvis. There are other ways to achieve this sensation, including Cat (p. 39) and Dog against the wall (p. 102). If Dog pose suits you, then enjoy it, but be sure to enter and leave slowly, keeping knees bent.

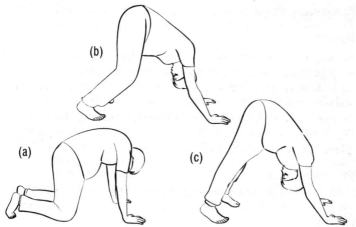

figure 3.21 a, b, c Cat–Dog–Cat

- Inhaling in Cat, keep lower back flat, knees hip width and hands strong.
- Exhaling, tuck in chin and tailbone to round spin.
- As exhale continues, maintain rounded back position, slowly lifting both knees from floor, keeping them bent.
- As exhale ends, sense you have lifted buttocks to a comfortable height.
- Inhale in Dog pose, keeping hands strong, shoulders wide and neck relaxed.
- If comfortable, straighten legs.
- Start exhaling, tuck in tailbone and chin to begin rounding spine.
- As exhale continues, lower both knees towards floor, keeping them bent.
- At end of exhale, return to rounded back Cat position.
- Inhale into flat back Cat.
- Exhale and rest in Hare pose (p. 40).
- Gauge your response and if comfortable then repeat up to five more rounds, either moving directly Cat–Dog–Cat and back to Dog, or resting in Hare pose between rounds.

Tips

If you are comfortable in Dog, remain for three rounds of breath, gently straightening and bending alternate knees.

Seated family

Restful, stabilizing and energizing.

Good strong, upright sitting posture is the foundation of many yoga practices, and can be easily achieved throughout pregnancy by judicious use of props. Once you have felt the strength, stability and peace of a secure sitting posture in yoga, it is easy to transfer the skills to achieve this in everyday life. Since so much time is spent sitting, whether in cars, whilst eating, watching television or working at computers, knowing how to sit strong and well can transform these everyday experiences into times of conscious awareness and postural improvement. With appropriate support, each of the seated poses also provides the base for a restorative pose.

Stick pose/Seated angle pose hybrid (dandasana/upavista konasana)

Usually in yoga, the legs in stick pose are touching, whilst in seated angle pose they are very wide apart. Neither of these options is comfortable or appropriate during pregnancy: the first provides no room for the bump, and the second can overstrain relaxed ligaments. This hybrid modification takes a middle path between two extremes. It develops strength in the spine whilst maintaining mobility in hips and legs, and is a valuable base position for many other practices, for example Energy freeing series (p. 120).

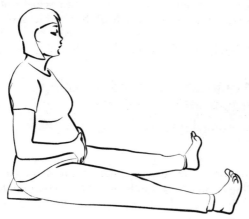

figure 3.22 Stick pose

- Use transitional moves (p. 27) down to floor.
- Stretch both legs out straight in front, wide enough apart to accommodate the belly easily.
- Flex both feet, pushing heels away and drawing toes backwards.
- Shift weight forward a little, and use hands to move buttock flesh diagonally out away from sitting bones. It should feel as if the pelvis tilts slightly forwards.
- Use hands on floor behind to provide support as needed.

Tips

Many pregnant women find that sitting flat on the floor exacerbates backache. To remedy this, use a small lift such as a block or cushion under the sitting bones to tilt pelvis and ease strain on lumbar spine. If backs of knees feel strained or uncomfortable with legs straight out, then place a cushion under knees.

Dandsasana can also be done against a wall to provide support. If your aim is to develop strength in the spinal muscles, or to use the pose for active rhythmic movements (pp. 55 and 57), then do it in the middle of the room. If your intention is to use the pose as a base position for breath, sound work, or meditative practices (Chapters 04, 05 and 06), then it can be more appropriate to sit against the wall.

To rest in this pose, place a chair in front and incline forwards, as in Restorative kneeling (p. 60). The chair seat front can be facing you, with your legs either side of the chair legs, or you can turn the chair sideways and rest on the side edge of the seat, with one of your legs between the chair legs.

Namaste quartet: four chest opening movements from stick pose

(These movements also work well from all other seated options in this section.)

Each movement in this sequence begins and ends with Namaste, the Indian palms-together greeting which signifies that our true understanding comes from the heart. This series mobilizes and strengthens the spine whilst opening the chest and deepening breath. The movements can be done independently, or as a flowing sequence. The key point is to synchronize breath and movement. To increase the focusing and stabilizing effects of the practices, put hands into Earth gesture (p. 21) as they move away from Namaste.

Namaste start and finish position

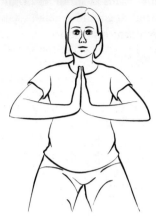

figure 3.23 Namaste quartet start/finish position

- Bring hands palms together in front of chest, fingers pointing up in Namaste.
- Inhale, exhale and push heels of hands together firmly.

Each part of this sequence begins and ends here. Unless otherwise mentioned, repeat each part up to ten rounds, synchronizing breath and movement.

Part one: open the heart

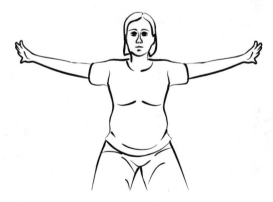

figure 3.24 Namaste quartet part one: open the heart

- Exhaling from start position, turn fingers to point out in front, straightening arms at shoulder height.
- Inhaling, open arms at shoulder height, as wide as possible.
- Exhaling, return to finish position.

Part two: lift the spirits

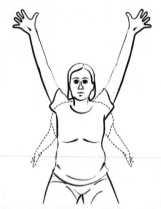

figure 3.25 Namaste quartet part two: lift the spirits

- Inhaling from start position, lift hands above head, separating them and opening arms to shoulder width, fingers spread wide.
- Exhaling, lower arms so fingertips touch floor behind you.
- Inhaling, reach arms back and out in a big circle until they reach above head.
- Exhaling, return to finish position.

Part three: reach with ease, a sideways stretch

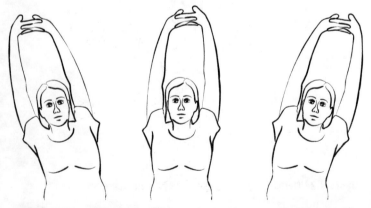

figure 3.26 Namaste quartet part three: reach with ease, a sideways stretch

- Inhaling from start position, reach hands above head and straighten arms back towards ears.
- Interlock fingers, and push palms up.
- Exhaling, ease over to right side, keeping both sides of torso long.
- Inhaling, return to centre.
- Exhaling, ease over to left side, keeping both sides of torso long.
- Repeat up to four rounds, synchronizing breath and movement.
- Exhaling, bring hands back to Namaste between rounds if you feel the need, returning to finish position at end of rounds.

Tips

Keep spine upright and long as you move from side to side. Hold arms well back and do not lean forward. It is better to limit the degree of side bend in the interests of maintaining an open chest. Once the movement is familiar, then focus equally on the contraction of the muscles on the side towards which you are leaning, and the stretch in the opposite side.

Part four: build vitality, an open twist

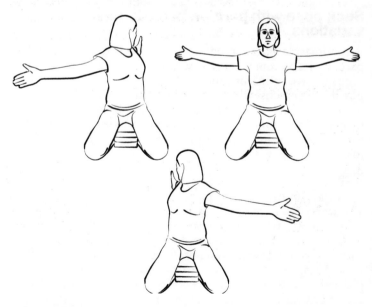

figure 3.27 Namaste quartet part four: build vitality, an open twist

- Inhaling, from start position, sit tall, extending arms to side at shoulder height.
- Exhaling, turn to right, moving from base of spine and stretching right arm out. Keep both shoulders low.
- Spiral twist through whole spine, until head turns and you can look over right shoulder.
- Inhaling, reverse movement, return to centre, bringing palms to Namaste.
- Repeat on other side.
- Alternate up to five rounds, synchronizing breath and movement.
- If movement feels comfortable, continue by remaining steady on each side for three rounds of breath, using inhale to lengthen spine and exhale to settle further into twist.
- Return to finish position.

Tips

Only take the twist as far as feels easy. In later pregnancy, you can acquire more space for the bump to turn by sitting raised on the edge of a block. Keep legs active and push into heels as you turn behind you. To deepen the focusing and stabilizing effects of the practice, put the hands in Earth gesture (p. 21).

Stick pose with partner: back-to-back variations

A comfortable variation on the Stick pose is to share it with a partner. To be comfortably sustainable, arrange the necessary props to give sufficient support. From this paired position it is possible to practise all the Namaste quartet variations above. Note that when your arms lift up, out and back, you are likely to come into contact with your partner's arms. With this variation, be aware of each other's comfort, and do not to turn too far into the twist.

Tips

This way your back is supported and sitting upright is easier. The warm presence of the partner also gives the advantage of being able to feel the movement of the breath in the partner's body (Entrainment breath, p. 157). If you discover that the curves of your two spines do not fit well, then put a flat cushion in between, behind either waist or shoulder blades. The precise placement of the cushion depends on the relative lengths and curves of your two spines, so experiment until it feels right.

Thunderbolt/Hero kneeling (vajrasana/virasana)

Thunderbolt and Hero are stable seats promoting a strong upright spine. Traditionally, vajrasana is practised by sitting back onto heels, keeping knees together, whilst virasana takes feet wider with buttocks down between heels. Both these classic poses fold calves and thighs tightly closed, which is often uncomfortable during pregnancy because the legs become heavier. Taking body weight straight down onto folded legs can exacerbate varicose veins. The following modifications render a hybrid version of these two valuable poses accessible and comfortable for practice during pregnancy by supporting upper body weight away from legs and feet.

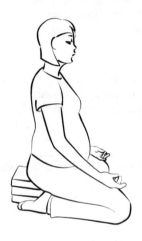

figure 3.28 Thunderbolt/Hero kneeling

- Place support (bolster, rolled blanket or yoga blocks) in middle of mat, narrow end facing front. The prop should be firm, stable and a minimum of 30 cm high to start.
- Follow transitional moves (p. 27) to all fours, placing middle of calves either side of front edge of prop.
- Walk hands towards knees and lower buttocks to sit on front edge of prop.

- Be upright, settling sitting bones firmly onto support and adjusting width of knees and feet until you feel secure.
- The pose should feel steady, and your lower back curve should be totally comfortable.

Tips

If you have it right, this pose should feel as if you could sit in it all day. If the lower back feels awkward, or you experience any discomfort in knees or ankles, adjust height of support. A sense of the lower spinal curve being 'jammed in', compression in knees or ankles, or overstretch in fronts of feet all indicate the need for higher support. A sense of being tipped too far forward indicates the need for lower support. The ideal height of support depends on many factors, including pelvic tilt, leg length and the size of your bump. It is worth keeping an open mind about the amount of support required, and adjusting it throughout pregnancy, since higher support is often more comfortable as the baby grows.

Vajrasana is the classic yoga after-dinner pose, recommended for ten minutes after eating to improve digestion. Once you have found a comfortable level of support in this kneeling seat, you can also use it as the starting point for the Hare pose forward resting (p. 40). Thunderbolt/Hero makes a stable base for Namaste quartet (p. 54) and is also an ideal seat for breath and sound work, energy practices and meditations (Chapters 04, 05 and 06).

Restorative kneeling

A sustainable kneeling seat is important for supported rest from Thunderbolt/Hero and is the basis for comfort in forward resting Hare pose (p. 40). In addition to the supported versions of Hare pose described above, more upright versions of this resting option include using a birthing ball or a chair for support. This base makes an excellent foundation for pelvic floor movements (p. 135) and many women find it helpful to use during labour (p. 200).

- Bring knees slightly wider than hip width apart, and provide padding if necessary before inclining spine forward.
- Relax shoulders as they rest on the support.

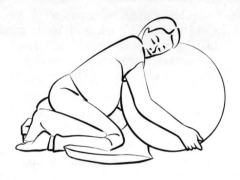

figure 3.29 Restorative kneeling with ball

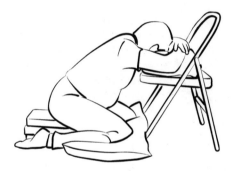

figure 3.30 Restorative kneeling with chair

Tips

The key to comfort in this pose is the correct height support. If the seat of the chair or the top of the ball is too low, then the lower back will tend to sag, making the pose uncomfortable. If you do not feel totally at ease, raise the height of support. If using a ball, make sure it is the right size. As a guide, women under about 165 cm are comfortable with birthing balls of 65 cm, and women over 165 cm need a ball sized 75 cm. These height guidelines also apply when sitting on the ball (p. 74).

Easy cross legs (sukhasana)

A steady base for the practice of Namaste quartet (p. 54), Energy freeing series (p. 120), and breath and meditation work (Chapters 04 and 05), this pose should feel spacious and sustainable. It strengthens the spine, enables you to breathe fully and freely, and brings good circulation to the pelvic organs.

Cautions

Keep legs free and open. Crossing them too tightly can exacerbate varicose veins and swollen joints. Usually in pregnancy it is more comfortable to use a cushion, block or other lift under the sitting bones to create an easy tilt in the pelvis. This provides more space for the growing bump and supports lower back curve.

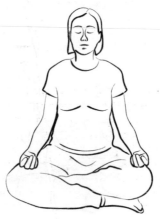

figure 3.31 Easy cross legs

- Use transitional movements to come to floor (p. 27) and sit with legs straight in front, hip width apart.
- Establish a full and easy rhythm of breath.
- Bend right knee and let it drop out to side.
- Bring right foot in front of pubic bone, with plenty of space (around 30 cm) between foot and perineum.
- Bend left knee and let it drop out to side.
- Cross left foot in front of right, so cross over point is about half way up shins.
- If using this seat for any longer than a minute or two, then swap cross of legs.

Tips

If your back gets tired or aches in this pose, then raise height of prop on which you are sitting, and/or place supports under knees. Sukhasana can also be used as a restorative pose, by placing a chair in front and inclining forwards as in Restorative kneeling (p. 60).

Sacral stabilizing/mobilizing seat (saithalyasana)

A hybrid modification of the previous cross-legged and kneeling seats, this pose has one leg in a variation of each position, providing a stable seated option which many women find very comfortable during pregnancy. It is also the basis of a Structural Yoga Therapy sequence specifically designed to mobilize and strengthen the lower back (p. 183). It is also, like all the other sitting bases, a good foundation for Namaste quartet (p. 54), Energy freeing series (p. 120) and breath and meditation practices.

Cautions

If you experience pain or stiffness in pelvic joints, this seat and the practices following may be a helpful remedy and future preventive, but approach with caution, since it is an asymmetrical base which can be tricky to achieve correctly at the start. If you do not feel stable on the floor, or if the pose causes discomfort in your ankles, knees or lower back, then sit on a fairly high support (a block or folded blanket under sitting bones) and gradually reduce height as your back and hips gain strength and mobility.

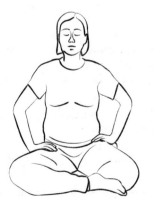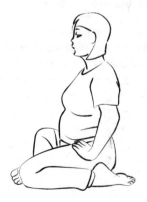

figure 3.32 Sacral seat (front and side)

- Use transitional moves (p. 27) to sit on floor with legs in front.
- Bend right knee and draw toes in to touch inside of left knee, allowing right knee to drop out sideways.
- Bend left knee up and take left foot to outer side of left buttock, so that front of left foot and ankle rest on floor, and toes of left foot point straight back behind you, tucked in towards side of left buttock.
- This is an uneven sitting base so weight will feel as if it is mostly on right sitting bone.
- To settle, circle pelvis gently five times in each direction before sitting tall and establishing an even breath.
- If using this seat as the basis for any other practices, reverse leg position half way through.

Sacral stabilization/mobilization sequence

This rhythmic sequence was devised by yoga therapist Mukunda Stiles to manage sacroiliac joint pain. To be most effective, it needs to be done in the order set out below. For comfort and ease in pregnancy, use props to sit on as described above.

This simple sequence is not only a powerful preventive of lower back pain, but can provide effective relief from existing discomfort.

Case study – Susan

I had experienced such severe pain in my lower back and hips on my previous pregnancies that I had been unable to walk for several weeks. It was awful. I was really worried the same thing would happen on this third pregnancy, but I found that if I practised this sequence every day I could manage the discomfort and relieve the pain almost completely. It was a revelation. To my great relief and surprise, I was able to be mobile and pretty much pain free throughout the whole pregnancy.

Part one: pelvic rocking

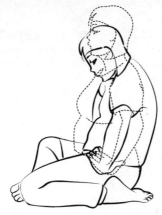

figure 3.33 Sacral sequence rocking forwards and backwards

- Be in sacral stabilizing seat (p. 63), with right foot in front and left foot tucked back behind, using whatever props are necessary for comfort.
- Place hands on hips, with fingers to front and thumbs pointing back in towards spine.
- Exhaling, tuck tailbone under, rounding spine backwards, as if fingertips were pressing back to tilt top of pelvis.
- Inhaling, reverse movement, lifting ribcage high and bringing curve of lower back forwards, as if thumbs were pressing pelvis forward and up.
- Alternate between these two movements, exhaling to round spine and inhaling as front of body lifts forward and up. Feel that the source of movement is the pelvis tilting.
- Repeat 14 times, or until movement feels smooth and easy, whichever takes longer.
- Move on to part two before switching leg position.

Part two: twisting

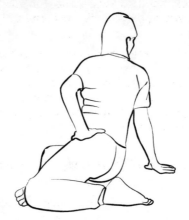

figure 3.34 Sacral sequence (twist)

- Be in sacral stabilizing seat (p. 63).
- Rest left hand on left hip.
- Inhaling, bring right hand to floor behind you and twist gently, opening chest, rolling left thigh inwards, and turning to look over right shoulder.
- Continuing to inhale, open chest and lean slightly into right hand so weight shifts more to right sitting bone and twist moves up spine. Be aware of muscles of left buttock engaging as left thigh is held in inward rotation.
- Exhaling, release twist and return to start position.
- Alternate between these two movements, inhaling as you twist and exhaling as you return. Feel that the source of movement is inward turning of left thigh which turns pelvis.
- Repeat 14 times, or until movement feels smooth and easy, whichever takes longer.
- Switch leg positions and return to repeat part one before repeating twists on other side.

Tips

The base position should be entirely comfortable before beginning the sequence. If you do not feel stable and secure, or if you sense any strain or pulling in the groin or knees, raise sitting bones higher, on a block or cushion. Pay attention to position of feet: toes of back foot should point backwards and not turn to side; toes of front foot should touch inside of opposite knee. If it is not easy for back hand to reach floor in the twists (for example if you are sitting on a block) then put a block on the floor under the hand.

For this sequence to build strength and support in the sacrum, it is important to feel which muscles are working to shift between the pairs of movements. In part one, whilst rocking pelvis, direct attention to buttock muscles close to sacrum in centre of lower back. In part two, focus interest in the strong contraction of buttock muscles closer to thigh as it turns.

Butterflies: half and full (ardha and purna titali asana baddokonasana)

These are comfortable seats for many women during pregnancy. With appropriate support (and the majority of pregnant women find the poses much more accessible with support as shown), they create ease in the lower back and spaciousness around the pelvis. They bring good circulation to pelvic organs and muscles of pelvic floor, and provide a secure base for other practices, including Namaste quartet (p. 54) and Energy freeing series (p. 120).

Cautions

If you experience discomfort in the pubic symphysis or pain in the sacrum, then either avoid these poses, or only practise with high support under sitting bones and thighs to reduce strain in pelvis.

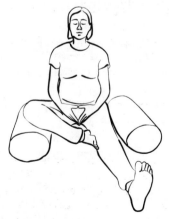

figure 3.35 Half butterfly with support

- Begin with sitting bones lifted on corner of a cushion or short edge of a block, to allow space for thighs to descend.
- Bring sole of right foot to inside of left thigh, allowing right knee and thigh to move out to side and down towards floor.
- Straighten left leg and push into left heel.
- Repeat on other side.

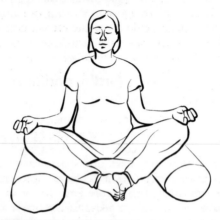

figure 3.36 Full butterfly with support

- Bring soles of feet together, allowing both knees to move out to side and thighs to move down towards floor.
- Adjust distance between heels and perineum until you feel a comfortable sense of openness through inner thighs.

In both full and half Butterflies:

- Use cushions or blankets to support back of thighs, about half way along thigh bone.
- Inhaling, sit tall, moving spine up away from pelvis.
- Exhaling, relax legs and pelvis into supports.
- Use each breath to settle more completely into pose, resting hands on knees or thighs in the gesture of your choice. Have elbows bent so upper arms drop down straight from shoulders, keeping chest open, and wrists and hands relaxed.
- If comfortable, focus on breath and remain in Butterfly for up to ten minutes or use it as a base for Namaste quartet or Energy freeing series.

Tips

If you experience any pulling or strain in thighs or pelvis, come out, and use Thunderbolt (p. 59) or Stick pose (p. 53) instead. The key to comfort in Butterfly during pregnancy is appropriate support. If you have to hold knees up, then strain in lower back results. Even (especially) if knees open easily right down to floor, use support as shown. The support enables weight of legs to release completely, removing any effort from the pose, and rendering it more sustainable and its many benefits more easily accessible. To rest in the pose, place a chair as for Restorative kneeling (p. 60). If you enjoy the openness of this pose and want to use it for a longer period, consider practising close to a wall for support from behind, or choose the restorative version pose described below.

Restorative butterfly/Golden womb rest (supta baddokonasana)

This is a blissful restorative pose giving complete support and protection to the back of the body to promote an attitude of receptivity, acceptance and contentment. It offers the essential openness of Butterfly, without physical effort. It can take a while to set up and uses lots of props but is well worth the effort because once you are in the pose, you can breathe, rest or do meditative practices in total comfort for up to 40 minutes or longer if you are comfortable. It is suitable for every stage of pregnancy.

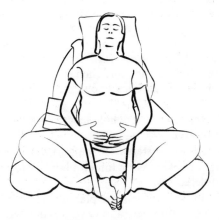

figure 3.37a Restorative butterfly (front)

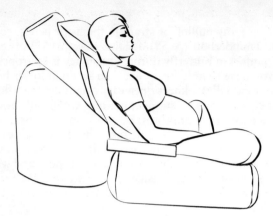

figure 3.37b Restorative butterfly (side)

- First assemble props: a mat, cushion or folded blanket to sit on, a belt to support sacrum, a bolster or two plus a wall or bean bag to provide inclined support, and bolsters or cushions for thighs and elbows. Additional cushions for head support can be useful, plus blanket and eyebag.
- Set up back support first, putting one end of bolster on cushion and leaning bolster against wall, using blocks, cushions or a bean bag to create a comfortable angle of around 30 degrees.
- Sit on cushion in front of bolster in full Butterfly (p. 68).
- Place belt around lower back, just below top rim of pelvis and bringing ends around to inside of your legs.
- Take belt underneath feet so that soles are held together without any effort. Adjust distance between heels and buttocks until it feels easy, and then secure belt to hold feet in this position. Place belt buckle so that it does not stick in your leg.
- Now lean back, ensuring whole length of spine is supported by upright bolster.
- Move cushions or bolsters in to support thighs and elbows.
- Use additional cushions or folded blankets to support head and neck if necessary.
- Cover with a blanket if you are planning to be in the pose for more than a few minutes, and cover eyelids with eye bag or scarf.

- Rest hands either on supports, or over your belly, whichever you prefer.
- Any core breath (Chapter 02), Heart/womb breath (p. 145), Inner silence meditation (p. 168) or yoga nidra (p. 166) are very beneficial this pose.
- When you feel ready to come out, move slowly and gently.
- First uncover yourself and draw knees inwards, supporting outside of knees with palms of hands.

Tips

When you recline, be especially attentive to supporting lower back curve, and if necessary, place an additional blanket at bottom of bolster. The final pose should create a feeling of complete support and comfort at all stages of pregnancy. If you are enjoying the pose, then there is no reason not to remain there for up to 40 minutes or more if you are still feeling comfortable.

Sitting with a chair

Sometimes it simply does not feel right to be sitting on the floor. It is helpful to have a repertoire of comfortable alternative sitting options.

Seated forward rest

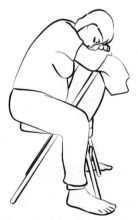

figure 3.38 Seated forward rest

- Choose a chair with a straight back, and a seat narrow enough to sit astride it.
- Check height of chair suits you: knees should be level with hips, or a little lower. If seat is too high, place blocks under feet to get properly grounded with heels on floor. If seat is too low, use blocks and/or cushions to raise it but make absolutely sure it is stable.
- Ensure feet, especially heels, are firmly down on floor.
- Moving from grounded sensation in the feet, pivot forward from hips and rest forearms on back of chair.
- Allow head to rest forehead down, or on one side.

Tips

This pose is a solid foundation for Namaste quartet (p. 54) or upper body section of Energy freeing series (p. 120).

Double chair extended forward rest

If you enjoy the forward rest option provided by a single chair, but require a longer reach (because of the size of your bump or the length of your legs and/or spine) then a second chair solves the problem.

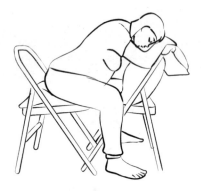

figure 3.39 Double chair extended forward rest

- Have two chairs with seats of equal height.
- Place second chair close to side of first chair, but only slide it into place after you are securely seated on first chair.
- Then, when front edges of two chair seats are touching, push back with your arms to slide buttocks onto second seat, thus extending reach of pose.

- Take feet as wide as comfortable, keeping heels well connected with floor.

Tips

This form of rest can be particularly useful in later pregnancy and in labour (p. 200).

Pelvic movement family

Relieving stiffness and pain in the lower back, promoting an energizing freedom of movement from body's core.

To a limited degree, this pelvic mobilization series can be done from any of the seated bases (pp. 52–72). They can be useful to free movement and relieve discomfort in any seated posture, for example on an office chair, or in an aeroplane, train or car seat. The full range of pelvic movements can also be done with great benefit from standing or squatting bases (pp. 79–96). In any position, the pelvic mobilization series is fabulous preparation for pelvic floor practices (p. 135). Additionally, these movements can also help to alleviate the acute pain of sciatica that may be encountered during pregnancy.

Case study – Madeleine

At around 33 weeks, I started experiencing stabs of sciatica in my left hip; yoga taught me easy ways to soothe those pains. I would heave myself out of bed, limp to the bathroom and spend about a minute rotating my hips as instructed: as if by magic, I could then walk normally again.

Ball and chair sitting

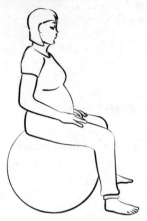

figure 3.40 Ball sitting

First choose a ball or chair the right height for you. Ideally when sitting with heels well grounded, knees should be about level with pelvis, or just a little lower. A 65 cm balls suit women around 165 cm tall, and taller women are more comfortable on 75 cm balls. With a chair, sit on a cushion to support the pelvic bones as you do the sequence described below. It is easier to get full mobility on a ball, but if you position yourself right at the front edge of a chair, then it is perfectly possible to move freely.

Pelvic tilting

- Keeping heels well grounded, establish a comfortable complete breath or Golden thread breath (p. 18).
- Rest hands on hips and tilt pelvis slowly forwards and backwards in time with breath.
- Inhaling, tilt forward, bringing weight onto pubic bone, arching lower back.
- Exhaling, tilt backwards, rounding lower back, bringing weight into base of sacrum, above coccyx (see Glossary).
- Repeat up to 11 times, or until movements feel smooth and easy.

Pelvic rocking

- Rock pelvis from right to left in time with breath.
- Inhaling, centre yourself, sitting tall and lifting ribs up out of pelvis.
- Exhaling, sink weight down into left sitting bone and heel, lifting right buttock slightly. Inhale back to centre.
- Exhaling, sink weight down into right sitting bone heel, lifting left buttock slightly. Inhale back to centre.
- Repeat rocking action up to eleven times, or until movements feel smooth and easy.

Pelvic circling and spiralling

This blends the two previous actions into a continuous fluid movement.

- Inhaling, tilt pelvis forward and shift weight down into right sitting bone and heel, slightly raising left buttock.
- Exhaling, tilt pelvis backwards and shift weight down into left sitting bone and heel, slightly raising right buttock.
- Return to centre and repeat, circling pelvis slowly and gently.
- Synchronize circles with breath rhythms; one half of circle matches inhale, and one matches exhale.
- Circle up to 11 times clockwise, then reverse and repeat in opposite direction.
- When you have a fluid ease with moving in circles, then improvise with spirals: allow circles to get progressively smaller, and then spiral out, allowing circles to grow progressively larger.

Tips

Keep feet, and especially heels, well grounded during these pelvic movements. Once these movements feel secure and familiar, then do the variations below.

The sequence in which these variations are presented provides a gentle progression to deeper release and increased mobility. The variations work especially well on a ball, but are also effective on a chair.

Pelvic spirals with arm sweeps

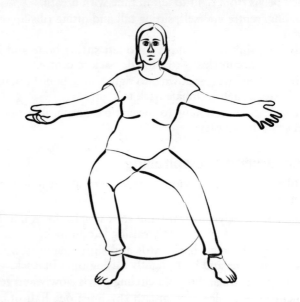

figure 3.41 Pelvic spirals with arm sweeps

- Sit steady, arms away from sides of body, palms backward.
- Inhaling, sweep arms back behind body.
- Exhaling, turn palms forward and sweep arms forward.
- After two or three arm sweeps, begin to circle pelvis clockwise.
- Synchronize rhythm of pelvic circles and arm sweeps with breath.
- After about 11 rounds in one direction, reverse direction of pelvic circles and repeat with arm sweeps.
- Lower arms and rest hands on hips.

Pelvic spiralling with eagle arms (garudasana)

This pose alleviates stiffness in upper back and shoulders, and promotes full chest breath.

- Sit steady, with feet grounded, hip width apart.
- Inhaling, bring elbows out to sides at just above shoulder height, forearms lifted at 90 degrees to upper arms.
- Exhaling, swing right elbow into centre, lining up vertical forearm with nose.

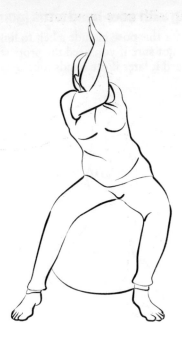

figure 3.42 Pelvic spiralling with eagle arms

- Settle with an inhale.
- Exhaling, swing left elbow into centre, crossing above right arm to hook left elbow up and over inner crook of right elbow.
- Wind arms together, catching left wrist with right hand.
- If this hold is easy, bring palms of hands together.
- Inhaling, lift elbows higher, keeping arms wound together.
- Exhaling, circle hips in whichever direction seems comfortable.
- Repeat for up to seven rounds of breath, each inhale lifting elbows and breathing into upper back, each exhale circling hips.
- To complete, stop pelvic circling, unwind hands and inhale to bring arms back out to side.
- Lower hands to hips and repeat, reversing cross of arms and changing direction of the pelvic circles.

This exercise can be varied by 'snaking' elbows in a side-to-side motion as they lift upwards whilst hips circle.

Pelvic spiralling with cow-head arms (gomukhasana)

The instructions for this pose include a belt to link right and left hands. If you are not sure if you need the prop, start out with it in place and discard it later if the hands touch.

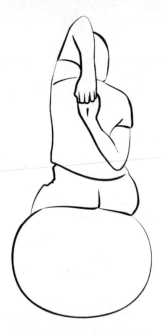

figure 3.43 Pelvic spiralling with cow-head arms

- Sit steady, feet grounded, hip width apart.
- Hold end of belt in left hand.
- Inhaling, reach left hand high above head.
- Exhaling, bend left elbow and let left hand dangle down back.
- Use right hand to cradle left elbow, gently moving it a little closer towards centre, behind head.
- Inhaling, swing right arm wide out to right side, and then reach it down and behind back, towards spine.
- Exhaling, bend right elbow and reach right hand up to take hold of dangling end of belt.
- With both hands on belt, inhale to open chest.
- Exhaling, work hands closer together. If hands easily move closely, then take hold of left hand with right and let go of belt.

- Begin to circle hips in whichever direction seems comfortable.
- Repeat for up to seven rounds of breath, each inhale breathing into sides of chest, and each exhale circling hips.
- To complete practice, stop pelvic circling, and unclasp hands.
- Lower hands to hips and repeat, reversing arm position and changing direction of pelvic circles.

Tips

Keep head aligned, and do not let upper arm push head and neck forward. Emphasize expansion of chest on inhalation and accompanying release that comes from pelvic circling.

Standing family

Strengthens back and legs, creating space and ease of motion in the spine.

Mountain pose (tadasana)

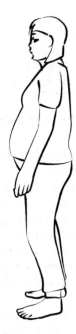

figure 3.44 Mountain pose (side)

This is a key posture in yoga, the pose whose alignment forms the basis of all standing postures. During pregnancy, as weight distribution and centre of gravity changes, it can be difficult to maintain comfortable and appropriate standing posture. Sometimes habitual ways of standing no longer feel easeful, or old injuries which you have long since forgotten begin to cause trouble. The softening of ligaments under the influence of pregnancy hormones can exacerbate these discomforts. Using the approach to standing described below can help you to discover a more gracious and easy posture to accommodate the changing shape and weight of the body throughout pregnancy and into the post-natal period.

- Stand with legs hip width apart, knees slightly bent and feet parallel. If this feels very peculiar, place feet as if they were the hands of a clock at about 'five-to-one', or 'ten-to-two'. Avoid turning toes out any wider than this, since outward rotation causes a duck waddle stance that can exacerbate lower back pain.
- Inhale up to top of lungs, lifting and opening front of chest and rolling shoulders back.
- Exhaling, let tops of shoulders drop and arms hang loose.
- Roll arms outwards and a little away from body so that palms face forward, giving more space to breathe into side ribs.
- Inhaling, spread toes wide apart from each other and take weight forward into balls of feet, lengthening neck and taking top of head upwards.
- Keeping knees bent, take weight right into pads of toes, starting with balls of feet and shifting weight through each toe pad in turn until it reaches little toes.
- Exhaling, roll weight to outside edges of feet and shift it back into heels as knees straighten.
- Keep arches of feet lifted and weight in heels for a moment, and then resume fluid shifting of weight around feet, bending knees and inhaling as weight moves forward into toes, and exhaling as it moves along outside edges of feet to drop into heels.
- When you feel ready, let weight settle naturally somewhere over centre of feet, keeping arches lifted.

Tips

Spinal curves alter during pregnancy, to bear the changing weight and shape of the growing bump. In this fluid version of the Mountain pose, be especially aware of curves of lower back and neck. Let the rolling action help you lengthen neck curve, by feeling the back of top of head rising upwards as weight drops. Let the dropping of the weight back into heels help you to lengthen lower back curve. Be aware of the relationship between these two curves, keeping chin parallel with floor and throat soft as lumbar curve lengthens.

Standing and walking pelvic scoops

Once you are familiar with the basic postural awareness of Tadasana, take it into daily life whenever you are standing or walking. The following wobbly walk is a transition between standing and walking that maximizes the mobility and strength of spinal curves.

- Use Tadasana described above as a base for pelvic tilting.
- Then turn tilt into a forward scoop, bending knees as tailbone moves forward, lengthening lower back curve.
- At end of scoop, straighten knees and return to start.
- Repeat up to ten times, progressively allowing effects of scoop to move up whole length of spine into neck and shoulders.
- Once scoops feel smooth, use it to carry a walk forward: lifting knee as tailbone scoops forward, and putting foot on floor at end of scoop.

Heavenly stretch

This uses Mountain pose as a base for an enlivening stretch, bringing freedom of movement along length of sides of body.

Cautions

With any pose that raises arms above head, changes in blood pressure occur. If you have low blood pressure, this can cause dizziness and/or fainting; if you have high blood pressure, you can feel uncomfortable and sense the heart beating very fast. If you encounter either of these experiences, do not raise arms higher than shoulder height, or keep arm movement fluid, for example not holding arms above head for more than a single inhalation and then lowering them. For most healthy pregnant women, this movement is completely comfortable and perfectly safe. It is pleasing (and less of a challenge to the heart) to do from any seated pose (pp. 52–3) as well as from standing.

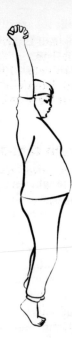

figure 3.45 Heavenly stretch (side, inhale)

- Stand in Mountain pose and breathe fully.
- Inhale, reach arms out to sides and above head, interlock fingers and straighten arms, reaching high. Push palms upwards.
- Exhale, bend elbows and rest hands on top of head.
- Inhaling, raise up onto balls of feet, reaching hands high.
- Exhaling, keep hands lifted high to maintain length in sides and back of body as heels descend.
- At end of exhalation, when heels are down, replace hands on top of head.
- Let breath move freely, reaching arms high on inhalation as heels lift, and lowering heels at end of exhalation.
- Repeat up to five more times, synchronizing each inhalation with upward reach and heel lift, and each exhalation with lowering of hands to top of head.
- To complete, exhale as arms lower to side and breathe steadily in Mountain pose for a few rounds.

Tips

If it is tiring to keep arms above head, then lower them to sides in between each round. If you feel an uncomfortably deep lower back curve as you raise up onto balls of feet, then keep knees slightly bent throughout and lengthen tailbone. To avoid wobbling, keep breath steady and eyes focused on a still point ahead of you.

Swaying palm tree (tiryaka tadasana)

A development from the previous pose, creating further freedom and mobility in the sides of the body, especially releasing space between bottom ribs and pelvic rim which often feels congested in pregnancy.

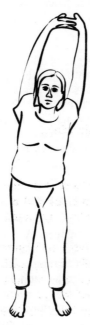

figure 3.46 Swaying palm tree

- Stand in Mountain pose and breathe fully.
- Inhale, reach arms above head.
- Exhale, interlock fingers and straighten arms, reaching high. Push palms upwards.
- Let breath move freely, reaching high on each inhalation and keeping heels well grounded on each exhalation.
- Inhaling, push right heel very firmly into floor and reach palms up, and then exhale and extend whole body over to left, keeping arms and trunk long.
- Inhaling, return to centre, and exhale to repeat on right side, keeping left heel grounded as body moves to right.
- Inhale and return to centre. Repeat three more times on alternate sides.
- To complete, exhale and lower arms to side, breathing steadily in Mountain pose for a few rounds.

Tips

If it is tiring to keep arms extended above head, then lower them to sides in between each round. Lift ribs up high out of pelvis to keep body long on both sides. The arms should be as far back behind head as is possible throughout. It is more important to maintain an open chest and length in sides of body than it is to move very far into sideways movement. Bring equal attention to contracting muscles on side towards which you are moving as to stretching muscles on long, open side of the body.

Footwork and balancing: arch strengthening

Often in pregnancy, lower back discomfort is accompanied by a slight collapsing of arches in feet. As ligaments soften, feet 'spread', and the resulting descent of the arches impacts directly upon support for the curves of the spine. Keeping feet strong and arches well lifted not only helps to support comfortable posture throughout pregnancy, it can help prevent swollen ankles too. The following sequence helps maintain healthy feet arches and provides support for strong and graceful standing posture throughout pregnancy.

Cautions

This variation, and indeed all balances in this section that bring weight onto one leg at a time, create an uneven load on the pelvis which can exacerbate pelvic pain. If you are experiencing pubis symphysis dysfunction, avoid standing on one leg for any of the following balancing practices and do not do these feet exercises from standing. Do them sitting down instead, from which position the pelvis will be supported symmetrically. If you have ever broken any of the bones in your feet, be especially gentle, and only bring a little weight down into the foot.

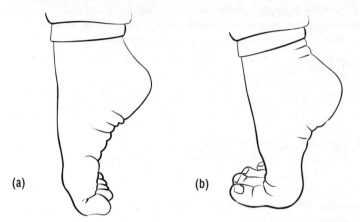

(a)　　　　　　　　　　(b)

figure 3.47 a, b Arch strengthening – toes tucked and heel lifted

Part one

- From standing, shift weight down into left foot.
- Inhaling, lift right heel and roll entire sole of right foot up away from floor until only tips of toes remain in contact with floor. Continue to raise heel until you can lightly tuck tips of all toes underneath, so nail sides of toes come into contact with floor.
- Exhaling, release and roll ball of foot back down to floor keeping heel lifted.
- Repeat up to seven times, rhythmically alternating the two positions in synchronization with breath.
- When movement feels smooth, move onto next part.

Part two

- From standing, keep weight shifted down into left foot.
- Inhaling, lift right heel and roll entire sole of right foot away from floor until only tips of toes remain in contact with floor.
- Exhaling, continue to raise heel until you can tuck tips of all toes underneath, so nail sides of toes come completely into contact with floor and front of foot is curved into an open stretch (figure 3.47a).

- Be sure every toe is tucked under. You may need to drop right knee out to side, if little toe is tricky to catch. Inhale.
- Keep foot in this position for a few rounds of breath, using exhale to take more weight down through foot into toes, breathing along curve of front of foot. Keep smiling.
- After a few rounds of breath release toes, bring weight back down into heel and move onto the next part.

Part three

- From standing, shift weight down into left foot.
- Inhaling, lift right heel and roll entire sole of right foot away from floor until only ball of the foot remains in contact with floor.
- Exhaling, spread toes very wide apart and press firmly into ball of foot as you keep heel raised up (figure 3.47b).
- Be sure pad of every toe is in contact with floor, and that equal weight is transferred down through each toe pad into floor. You may need to drop right knee out to side if little toe does not feel engaged.
- Breathe easily with foot in this position, using each exhale to take more weight down through ball of foot into toes. Keep smiling, and keep heel well lifted.
- After a few rounds of breath, release position, keep weight balanced in left foot and shake out right foot, starting at toes, and working up through ankle, knee, thigh and buttock until you can shake whole leg out with a little kick from hip to toes.
- Once you have shaken out leg, place right foot back on floor and notice the different sensations between left and right foot. Then repeat all three parts of series on other side.

Tips

This practice brings energy through feet up into legs and pelvis. It enlivens standing posture and boosts vitality. Go gently, since over-enthusiastic practice can cause cramp. Pace yourself and feel how much weight you can comfortably take down through feet in parts two and three. As you increase this gradually, smile softly and explore your response to the minor physical discomfort the pose can create.

Tree balance (vrksasana)

The foot exercises described above are an excellent preparation for balancing practices.

Cautions

As for all one-legged balances (p. 84)

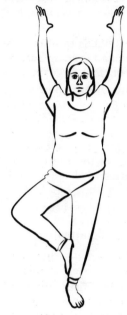

figure 3.48 Tree balance

- Stand in Mountain pose (p. 79), with feet parallel and legs hip width apart.
- Bring palms together in Namaste.
- Breathe fully, carrying awareness from heels to top of head on inhalation, and back down to heels on exhalation.
- Focus eyes on a still point straight ahead and, exhaling, slowly shift weight into left foot.
- Inhaling, bend right knee and slowly lift right foot away from ground, heel first.
- Exhaling, ground balance through left foot, lifting right knee up in front, and turn it out to side.

- Allow sole of right foot to come to rest on inside of left leg, just below knee. Continue to breathe freely and easily.
- When you feel steady and balanced, slowly raise joined palms straight up in front of face and over head, opening out arms once hands reach top of head.
- In final pose, let arms be as wide as comfortable to allow tops of shoulders to relax down away from ears and chest to feel open. Take a few rounds of breath here, keeping eyes focused steady.
- To descend, first lower hands to heart. Then release sole of foot from inside of leg, and keeping knee lifted, bring it back to centre before lowering foot to ground.
- Stand for a few rounds of breath in Mountain pose before repeating on other side.

Tips

Physical balance in this pose depends upon breath awareness and visual focus, so do not to rush into physical movement before eyes and breath are settled. If you find it easy to balance with foot below knee, then draw foot higher up to rest against thigh. Avoid letting sole of foot rest against inside of knee, since this can cause strain. If you lift foot higher than knee, ensure pelvis still faces forward. Be attentive to lower back curve, keeping it long and easy.

T-shaped balance/Modified warrior 3 (Virabhadrasana 3)

Strictly speaking, this pose is part of the family of warrior stance postures (p. 104), but is included here because essentially it is an open balance. If you feel poised and steady in the previous poses, then this balance can be especially enjoyable in pregnancy, especially if you need to reclaim some more space and length in the body as the bump grows.

Cautions

As for all one-legged balances (p. 84).

If you experience pelvic pain, avoid this asana and replace with Dog against the wall for a similar effect (p. 102).

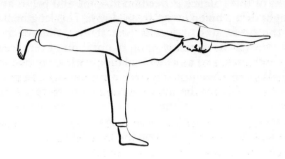

figure 3.49 T-shaped balance

- Begin in Mountain pose, feet parallel and hip width apart. Inhale.
- Exhale, and step left leg forward, keeping knee bent and grounding weight through left foot.
- Inhale, stretch arms straight out in front and up above head at shoulder width, straightening elbows.
- Exhaling, reach forward with arms and torso, slowly raising right leg off floor behind you, keeping foot flexed.
- Keep eyes focused on a still point straight ahead as you breathe evenly and come to a place of steadiness where left leg raises towards hip height (no higher) and head and neck settle in between upper arms (no higher).
- With each inhalation, extend length through back of body, from fingertips to heel.
- With each exhalation, deepen foundation of balance by pressing left heel into floor, keeping arch of foot lifted. If you wish, straighten left leg, but if you sense this compromises your balance, let it remain bent.
- Take one or two rounds of breath, and then inhale as you slowly reach arms and torso forwards and upright, lowering right foot to floor.
- Exhale and lower arms.
- Breathe for a couple of rounds in Mountain pose and repeat on other side once or twice more.
- At end of balance, rest in Mountain pose/Ladder against wall (p. 98) or transition down to floor to Hare pose (p. 40).

Tips

The delight of this balance is freedom in spine and pelvis as the entire weight of the bump hangs freely down. This lengthens the back of the body, and it works best if you can reach far forwards. Steadiness depends upon maintaining even breath, still focus with eyes, and a firm foundation with grounded foot. Because balance in this pose improves very rapidly and readily with repetition, it can be an encouraging posture to build security and confidence in the abilities of the pregnant body. Appropriate cautions permitting (see p. 84), this balance can be practised right through to late stages of pregnancy.

Squatting family

Builds leg strength, boosts pelvic circulation and enables you to discover your own comfortable open pelvis position for birth.

Partial and supported squats can be strengthening and energizing throughout pregnancy. They promote a deep connection with the earth element, both physically and energetically, and can be helpful in the prevention and relief of upper and lower back pain. All the poses in this section are based on a squatting action. There is no need to squat deeply, shallow dips work just as well.

Cautions

Keep your feet well grounded and only descend in any squat as far as you can manage easily without your heels rising from floor. If you have a history of prolapse, or injuries to your knees and/or lower back, do only supported squats and descend only slightly.

Supported squat/Fierce pose modification (utkatasana)

This is the safest and most accessible way to enjoy squatting during pregnancy. Even if you think you cannot squat, this method gives easy access to the pose. Your partner does not have to be the same height as you.

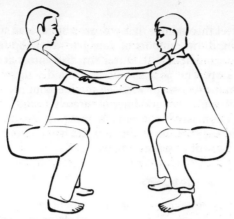

figure 3.50 Supported squat

- Stand in Mountain pose, about arm's length away from your partner.
- Take your legs slightly wider then hips (about yoga mat width is a good guide), bend knees very slightly and have feet either parallel or slightly turned out.
- Each partner takes a firm grasp of the other's forearms and straightens the arms.
- Step back if necessary, so that straightening arms causes upper back to round. Upper back should feel open and stretched so each partner can lean their weight back, trusting the hold of their partner.
- Inhale as you alternately pull forward and back on each arm, dropping shoulders and bringing a soft rhythmic twist into upper back.
- Exhale, push into heels and move buttocks out behind, tucking tailbone under to round out lower back curve.
- Whole of spine should feel in a comfortable curve.
- Exhaling, bend knees deeper, keeping lower back rounded and a strong sense of support in upper back as you lean back against your partner's weight.
- Descend on exhale only so far as you can comfortably go with heels remaining in firm contact with floor.
- Inhale and straighten knees to ascend.
- Repeat up to five times, exhaling down and inhaling up. Take pauses between rounds if that feels more comfortable.

Tips

You should feel throughout that you are able to lean well back, totally trusting in the support of your partner. Keep feet active and engaged throughout. If you feel any discomfort at all in the lower back, stop. The pose should create a delightful sense of easy release in the whole spine. Once you feel comfortable doing this squat with a partner, and have accurately gauged the degree of descent appropriate for you, then experiment with different forms of solid support, for example a kitchen counter top, low table, or the back of a (secure) chair.

Squatting namaskaram

This standing sequence adapts the opening invocation of classical Indian dance (Bharatanatyam). It promotes graceful posture and elegant fluid movement whilst energizing the whole body. In late pregnancy the stamping of the feet can also send a message to the baby within that you are ready for their arrival.

Cautions

The alternate stamps can exacerbate pelvic pain, so if you are experiencing public symphysis dysfunction, replace stamps with pelvic circles and tilts.

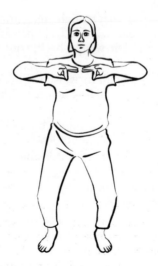

figure 3.51 Squatting namaskaram basic

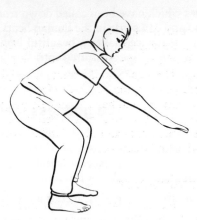

figure 3.52 Squatting namaskaram forward reach

- Stand in Mountain pose with legs as wide apart as is comfortable for the squat described above.
- Inhaling, bend elbows out to sides, resting hands in front of heart in Earth gesture (p. 21).
- Exhaling, sink as deep as comfortable into squat (figure 3.51).
- Inhaling, keep hips and pelvis steady by tightening buttocks as you stamp right foot to floor.
- Exhaling, repeat with left foot, and then twice more, alternating right and left.
- Inhale, return to standing in steady squat and exhale into a forward reach, taking buttocks out well behind you and opening fingers wide with hands palms down to offer a blessing to the earth (figure 3.52).
- Inhale, circle arms wide around, bringing them above head.
- Exhaling stand upright, bringing hands back to heart in Earth gesture.
- Repeat up to three times.

Tips

The sequence has a powerful symbolism with which many women connect very deeply in pregnancy. The stamping feet call the heavens to earth, in the same way as the child's spirit is called into a human body in the mother's womb. The forward reach with open palms offers thanks and blessing to the earth, asking for her forgiveness for having stamped upon her; and the final circling of the arms and return to the heart signifies that the heavenly energies which have been called down from above now reside all around and can settle in the human heart and bless the child within. The sequence makes a beautiful beginning to any yoga practice, or can be incorporated into flowing sequences (p. 177).

Victory pose of the fierce goddess (devijai utkatasana)

This asana is an energizing expression of the creative force of feminine energy that manifests especially fully in pregnancy. The 'face pulling' element also makes it fun to do.

- Stand in Mountain pose (p. 79), feet at a comfortable width for squatting.
- Have feet parallel, or slightly turned out and hands at heart in Namaste.
- Inhale, straighten legs, raising arms up straight above head, wider than shoulders, with fingers spread wide.
- Exhale loudly through mouth, bend knees and elbows to drop straight down towards earth.
- On descent, stick out tongue as far as it will go and roll eyes up and back.
- At end of exhale, return to start position.

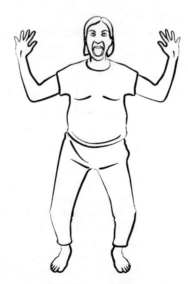

figure 3.53 Victory pose of the fierce goddess

Tips

The louder the exhale, the more energizing the pose. Stick your tongue right out and widen your eyes as you roll them back. Be cautious about lower back curve as you descend: it should feel comfortable and easy. Bend knees on descent and keep weight down in heels to avoid compressing lumbar vertebrae.

Lord of the dance (natarajasana II)

This elegant open balance pairs very well with the previous pose: alternating between them makes a pleasing contrast between the earthy descent of Fierce goddess and the spacious airy poise of Lord of the dance. The combination works best if the Fierce goddess pose comes between left and right side balances of Lord of the dance.

Cautions

As for all one-legged balances (p. 84).

If you are experiencing pubic symphysis dysfunction or sacroiliac pain, then keep both feet on the floor in this pose, and just do the squatting with arm moves.

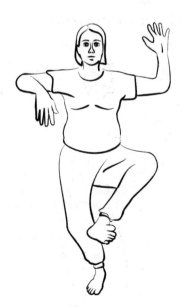

figure 3.54 Lord of the dance

- Stand in Mountain pose, feet at a comfortable width for squatting.
- Inhale taking elbows wide to side at shoulder height.
- Exhale and drop deeper into squat, taking weight into right foot.
- Inhale and raise left leg, taking left knee to side and lifting left foot to bring shin towards horizontal at knee height.
- Keep breath even as you balance with elbows wide, raising left hand to push palm fowards, fingers pointing up.
- Let right wrist bend, and fingers of right hand point down towards earth.
- Exhaling, release hand positions, keeping elbows out to side and bringing left foot back to ground, returning to squat.
- Inhale, and repeat on other side.
- Repeat up to five times, alternating between left and right sides and synchronizing movement with breath.
- Return to Mountain pose for a few rounds of breath.

Tips

If you get confused about coordination, remember that the lifted hand corresponds to the lifted leg. Keep transitions between one side and the other smooth and even. The experience of balance and poise is more secure if you keep eyes focused on a still point ahead of you. Being mindful of the meaning of the gestures deepens your experience of the pose: the raised hand with palm forward signifies 'fear not', whilst the fingers pointing to the earth draws attention to the ground of our being and the need for a down-to-earth connection even as we dance in the air. These attitudes of courage and earthiness are especially valuable to cultivate during pregnancy as preparation for childbirth and motherhood.

Wall supported family

Offering a unique combination of resting and strengthening options to improve posture and build strength in supported poses.

The postures in this family can help you to prevent back pain, but may also be used for relief of discomfort.

Case study – Lisa

Doing the yoga stretching helped significantly with the recurring upper back pain I experienced in my first pregnancy. The weekly classes totally alleviated the pain each week and showed me moves that I could use at home to relax my back. The most useful series were the ones against the wall.

A wall (or closed door, or broad tree trunk) is a helpful support for the upright spine in the full range of sitting poses (pp. 52–73). In particular, the addition of a cushion under the buttocks and a flat pillow behind the lower back can make wall-supported stick pose, Butterfly and Easy cross-legged seats into sustainable postures for meditations (see Chapters 05 and 06) and breathwork (see Chapters 02 and 04).

The wall is also a useful support for the following standing postures. This family of active and resting poses are very helpful throughout pregnancy to maintain (or discover) postural awareness that can lead to more comfortable alignment, creating length and strength through the spine. This group works well as a coherent series, but each pose can also be done in conjunction with other base positions, for example, using Chair and Side Stretch against wall as preparation for poses in the Cat family (all fours) (p. 38), or Dog against wall as a preparation for flowing sequences (p. 177).

Ladder against wall (modified upright advasana/reversed corpse pose)

This upright resting option uses the wall for support, comfort and privacy. It is an upright version of the horizontal rest on the front of body, which many pregnant women (especially if you enjoyed sleeping on your front before pregnancy) particularly enjoy as a replacement for front-lying postures. It makes a comfortable base for various modified upright resting positions during first stage labour (p. 200).

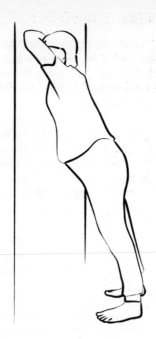

figure 3.55 Ladder against wall

- Stand in Mountain pose, about 50 cm away from wall, with feet hip width apart and parallel.
- Inhale and reach arms up above head, palms facing the wall.
- Exhale, shift weight into balls of feet, tilting body forwards until hands and arms come into contact with wall.
- Bend arms, catch each elbow with opposite hand, and rest head on forearms.
- Breathe fully, sweeping mental awareness from heels to head on inhale, and from head to heels on exhale.
- Settling into pose, creep elbows higher up wall to bring length and space into sides of body.
- Rest here as long as you need, and then follow with next pose.

Chair against wall (modified fierce pose/utkatasana)

This is a useful pose for checking the changing curves of the spine during pregnancy. It can help to relieve lower backache, counteract stooping shoulders and strengthen lower back, feet and legs.

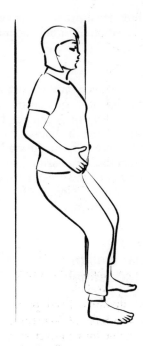

figure 3.56 Chair against wall

- Stand in Mountain pose, with your back about 50 cm away from wall.
- Feet parallel, hip width apart, arches well lifted.
- Inhale, reach back to bring palms of hands flat on wall.
- Exhale, let arms take weight of body as you slowly ease spine to wall. When spine is resting against wall, bring palms together on chest in Namaste.
- Inhale and lengthen spine, keeping tailbone, head and shoulder blades in contact with wall.
- Exhale, press palms together and bend knees slightly, sliding spine a little down wall.

- Inhale and arch lower back a little away from wall whilst maintaining contact between back of head and wall.
- Exhale and lengthen curve of lower back, bringing it closer to wall and squeezing buttocks together.
- Keep feet strong, arches lifted, and breath flowing freely as you continue to tilt pelvis in time with breath for up to seven or eight rounds.
- To complete, straighten legs, press palms against wall and push back to starting position. Rest in Ladder against wall for a few rounds of breath.

Tips

Bend knees only slightly, and slide only a short way down wall; emphasis is upon spinal alignment, not causing strain in thighs and knees. Up to about 30 weeks of pregnancy, the pelvic tilting will probably enable you to bring the lumbar curve into contact with wall. As lower back curve deepens during later pregnancy, this is not always comfortable or possible, so bring palms of hands onto wall, one on top of the other, at about waist level, resting lower back curve against back of top hand. If this support is too deep, then just use one hand and rest other hand on belly.

Side stretch against wall (modified swaying palm tree/tiryaka tadasana)

The best pose for creating space and openness along sides of body.

- Stand in Mountain pose, with right side about arm's length from wall, feet parallel, hip width apart.
- Inhale, raising right hand to shoulder height and press palm into wall. If necessary, adjust distance from wall so that right arm can be held straight at shoulder height.
- Exhale and push back of left heel firmly into floor.
- Inhaling, raise left arm above head, with elbow straight or bent.
- Exhale, push right palm into wall and heel of left foot firmly down into floor, letting head and neck tilt slightly to right and feeling descent of left heel freeing movement through left side of body.
- Inhale, breathe fully into open space around left armpit and ribs.
- With each inhalation, reach left arm higher up.
- With each exhalation, press right palm firmly against wall and left heel down into ground.

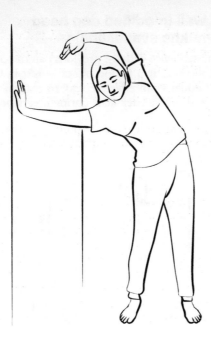

figure 3.57 Side stretch against wall

- Continue for up to five rounds.
- To come out, inhale right arm back up above head, and exhale both arms down to sides.
- Pause for a round of breath in Mountain pose before reversing position to repeat on other side.

Tips

Keep arm which presses against wall completely straight at shoulder height, because it is the direct pressure from this arm, moving across the chest, which opens space between ribs on opposite side. When you can feel the movement coming under the raised arm, between each rib, then lung function is improved by providing more space. This sideways expansion is especially important in pregnancy, as the lungs have less room, and the movement of the respiratory diaphragm is limited as the baby grows. For this reason, enhancing your capacity to expand the breath into sides and back of ribs is an effective way to reduce breathlessness and boost vitality.

Dog against wall (modified dog head down/adho mukha svanasana)

This works well in sequence with the previous pair of poses. Three rounds of Dog followed by a period of active rest in Chair and recuperation in Ladder is an effective way to realign the spine, improve posture and relieve back ache during pregnancy.

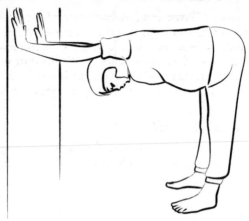

figure 3.58 Dog against wall

- Stand in Mountain pose, facing wall at arm's length distance.
- Inhaling, reach arms above head to place palms on wall, shoulder width apart.
- Exhaling, press weight into heels, keeping arches lifted.
- Keeping breath even, slowly walk palms of hands down wall, no lower than hip height.
- Step feet back away from wall little by little to create length in spine. Move only as far away as enables you to keep hips straight above ankles, with strong hand contact on wall. Do not step further back than this.
- Keep feet hip width apart and parallel, arches lifted and weight pushing down into heels.
- Spread fingers wide and keep strong pressure from heels of hands into wall.
- Inhaling, lengthen sides of body, pushing heels of hands into wall.
- Exhaling, lengthen spine towards tailbone, pushing heels of feet into floor.

- Breathe here up to five rounds.
- To come out, slowly walk hands up wall and step feet in towards wall.
- Rest for a few rounds of breath in Ladder against wall (p. 98).
- If you enjoyed the pose, repeat twice more.

Tips

Only walk hands down and feet back away from wall as far as you feel secure. If you experience any discomfort in the lower back, bend the knees. Once you have a secure foundation, then use Mountain pose feet movements (p. 80) to shift weight, and pelvic tilts and circles (p. 81) to mobilize lower back. Enjoy the freedom in the pelvis as the weight of your belly hangs forward.

Warrior against wall

An excellent preventive and relief for calf cramps, this also makes perfect preparation for the family of Warrior poses which follow.

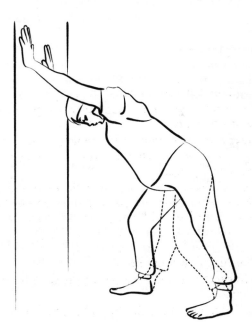

figure 3.59 Warrior against wall

- Follow instructions for Dog against wall (p. 102) until you come to a sustainable posture which you can maintain with comfort and security for a couple of minutes. If necessary have hands higher up wall than for previous pose.
- Let breath move freely and easily.
- Keeping feet hip width apart, step right foot forwards, far enough to enable right knee to bend without it moving forward of right ankle. Keep left leg straight.
- Exhaling, shift weight from one foot to the other, and pivot on left heel to turn left foot out slightly if it feels more comfortable.
- Inhaling, press heels of hands into wall.
- Exhaling, press outside of left heel into floor, keeping leg straight and carrying mental awareness down through calf muscles.
- If you are comfortable, stay for up to a minute or two, keeping a rhythmic flow of breath and awareness through left leg, pressing heels of hands against the walls on inhale and heels of feet, in particular left heel, against floor on exhale.
- Keeping feet in same positions, bend left knee and straighten right leg.
- Continue for up to a minute or two with same rhythmic breath and mental awareness used for first position.
- Rest in Ladder against wall (p. 98) for a few rounds of breath and repeat with left foot forwards.

Warrior family

Working from the ground up to encourage good posture, stamina and freedom of breath and energy.

A pregnant warrior is an alarming concept, a contradiction in terms. Yet many qualities promoted by the series of yoga poses known as 'warriors' are of great value during pregnancy. Their practice promotes stability, resilience, courage and strength. Classic warrior form often requires a stride so wide that it can strain the vulnerable ligaments of the pregnant body, bringing pressure into pelvic floor and lower back. But these adapted variations enable you to benefit from the essential qualities of the poses without unnecessary strain.

Basic adapted warrior stance for pregnancy

In contrast to the classic wide-legged warrior stance, this pregnancy modification uses a shorter stride and softens the pose, giving the option to shift from bent knee to straight as you need. Use this base for the four poses which follow.

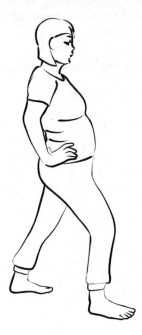

figure 3.60 Basic adapted warrior stance

- Stand at front of mat, legs about hip width apart and feet parallel.
- Bend knees, let shoulders and heels drop.
- Breathe fully, bringing palms together at chest.
- Exhaling, step left foot backwards, maintaining hip width between legs and only taking a short stride.
- To begin, have right knee slightly bent, and left leg straight.
- Pivot on ball of left foot to angle toes out slightly to right, keeping arches lifted.
- Inhale, lengthen back of body from left heel through to top of head.
- Exhale, feel weight descending through both heels.

- Settling in pose, experiment with weight distribution by alternately bending and straightening right knee. If necessary adjust length of stride slightly to accommodate shifting weight.
- To come out, inhale and step left foot forward, returning to Mountain pose.
- Breathe a few rounds here before repeating on other side, stepping back with right foot.

First warrior adaptation (Virabhadrasana 1)

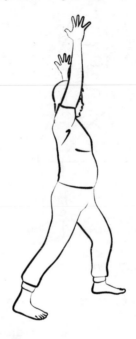

figure 3.61 First warrior adaptation

- Begin in Basic adapted warrior stance, left leg forward, knee bent.
- Inhaling, stretch arms out to sides and above head at shoulder width, spreading fingers wide.
- Exhaling, drop shoulders and press back of right heel and outside of left foot down into mat.

- With each inhale, reach up through arms, lifting ribs away from pelvis which remains square and forward, facing over left knee.
- With each exhale, sink weight down through heels of feet, keeping back leg strong and straight.
- Breathe here for up to five rounds before lowering arms and returning to Mountain pose.
- Reverse leg position and repeat on other side.

Second warrior adaptation (Virabhadrasana 2)

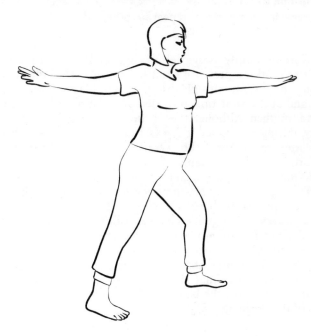

figure 3.62 Second warrior adaptation

- Begin in basic adapted warrior stance, left leg forward, knee bent.
- Inhaling, stretch arms out to sides and above head at shoulder width, spreading fingers wide.
- Exhaling, drop shoulders, taking arms down to form horizontal line at shoulder height, palms face down.

- Inhaling, broaden chest by taking arms wide. Turn upper body to right, reaching right arm out behind and left arm out in front over knee.
- Exhaling, press back of right heel and outside of left foot down into ground.
- With each inhale, reach out through arms, lifting ribs away from pelvis which remains facing right.
- With each exhale, sink weight down through heels, keeping back leg strong and straight.
- Breathe here for up to five rounds before lowering arms and returning to Mountain pose.
- Reverse leg position and repeat on other side.

Tips

For Warrior family poses let ribcage and spine lift up on inhalation, taking pressure from lower back. Keeping strong pressure down into straight back leg will help to ground the pose, and at the same time provide a foundation from which to lift and lengthen. Although these poses are usually held firm and steady, during pregnancy it can feel more appropriate to bring fluid movement into the Warrior poses to keep them comfortable and sustainable. Do this by rocking weight from foot to foot, shifting the bend in the knee from front leg to back leg, circling, tilting and scooping the pelvis to lengthen lumbar curve. It can also be beneficial to shift from First warrior to Second warrior in a gentle rhythm following the breath, for example, inhaling up into First warrior, and then exhaling arms to side and inhaling around into Second warrior, and back again. These rhythmic shifts in upper body position can be accompanied with knee bends, creating a soft cycle of movements that free the basic pose to better accommodate the needs of the pregnant body.

Warrior of the heart (adapted upright parsvottanasana)

The most powerful warrior of all, this pose promotes courage and fearless acceptance by opening the heart. In images of the goddess at her most triumphant, her hands are empty, since she is understood to have defeated her enemies and have no further need of weaponry. As in this pose, her strength comes from within.

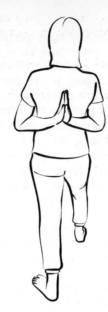

figure 3.63 Warrior of the heart

- Begin in basic adapted warrior stance, right leg forward, knee bent.
- Breathe fully, pushing heels into mat.
- Inhaling, raise both arms out to side at shoulder height.
- Exhaling, slide shoulder blades down and bring arms behind back, catching hold of each elbow with opposite hand.
- Take a full round of breath in this hold, gauging your comfort level.
- If shoulders and arms are comfortable, then slowly bring palms together behind back. If this causes discomfort, return to previous hold.
- Let tailbone drop and circle pelvis gently as you breathe into open chest for up to five rounds.
- With each inhale, open chest and lengthen upper body, moving up and out of pelvis.
- With each exhale, sink weight down through heels of feet, keeping back leg strong and straight.
- Release hand hold, lower arms and return to Mountain pose.
- Breathe for a few rounds, then reverse leg position and repeat on other side.

Tips

The tendency in this pose is to open the front of the body at the expense of letting your lower back curve collapse inwards. To avoid this, lift upper body away from pelvis, and engage buttock muscles strongly to support lower back. Be aware of the symbolism of the pose: that a truly open heart is a source of such courage and confidence that we need no weapons to protect ourselves; the solid support for the open heart comes from the strength of the body behind. We can face every challenge with composure and acceptance because we feel fully grounded and supported. This attitude is especially valuable to cultivate on the journey of pregnancy that leads through the challenge of childbirth into the adventure of motherhood.

04

the energy body: water

In this chapter you will learn:
- breath patterns to relieve anxiety and promote contentment
- yoga remedies for erratic energy and disturbances to the nervous system
- combined pelvic floor and breath practices to create stability, increase energy and improve posture.

Water gesture (apas/varuna mudra)

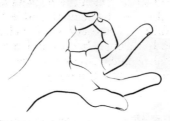

figure 4.1 Water gesture

With hands resting palms up, comfortably on knees or thighs, lightly touch tip of little finger to tip of thumb. The other fingers are relaxed. This hand gesture connects to the energy of the water element, enhancing qualities of fluidity, movement and adaptability. The gesture can be used together with the core breaths and/or the postures described in the previous two chapters, or with the movement and breath practices described in this chapter. It is also useful when you sense that the flow of energy in your body is blocked, for example if you feel sluggish, overtired, or so fizzing with nervous energy that you cannot sleep.

Yoga perspectives on energy

The name for energy or life force in yoga is 'prana'. The term describing the energy body is 'pranamaya kosha', and the word 'pranayama' describes any practices which alter the flow of prana in the body, for example everything in this chapter. In yogic understanding, the energy body is linked with the water element because currents of prana are said to flow like water in channels and streams throughout and beyond the physical body, both pervading and surrounding it. The pathways of these many thousands of currents are called 'nadis', which is Sanskrit for 'river', and the connection between physical and pranic (energy) bodies can helpfully be compared to the relationship between earth and water: the land is irrigated and nourished by the waters flowing through it, and rivers and streams carry in their waters the traces of the earth through which they flow. So too, the energy body brings life and vitality to the physical body, whilst currents and movements of prana are influenced by the characteristics of the 'earth', the physical body, through which they flow. The extent to which these rivers of energy are also influenced and directed by mental and emotional states is explored more fully in Chapter 05. This chapter works with energy in the body through breath and movement practices which boost vitality and promote a free flow of energetic currents throughout the physical body.

Changes to the energy body in pregnancy

Support for a woman's experience of pregnancy is often focused upon her physical body: there are scans to monitor the baby's growth, and blood and urine tests to check the changing biochemistry of pregnant bodily systems; the growing bump is palpated and measured by midwives, whilst well-meaning friends, relatives and sometimes strangers feel free to offer constant comments about its shape, size and form. But whilst these physical alterations are the most publicly visible and easiest to detect, it is often changes to the energy body which have the most significant impact upon a pregnant woman's daily life.

The very deep levels of exhaustion, for example, which so often accompany the first 18 weeks of pregnancy, can be more vivid to a busy woman than any amount of information about the fabulous developments of the baby within: all she knows is that she is falling asleep at lunchtime and snoring on the sofa before she's had a chance to cook any supper. The volatile shifts in vitality that can occur in the second trimester of pregnancy, once the placenta is fully formed and functioning, provide a bumpy ride for the woman who finds herself pacing the house at two in the morning, writing endless lists of things to do, imagining future plans for her baby, and worrying about how she is going to make it through the next day on two hours of sleep. Once the pregnancy is reaching its end, and managing the physical challenge of the fully grown bump may have become second nature, then surprising waves of powerful nesting energy may prompt many a previously undomesticated woman to embark on ambitious cleaning and clear-out campaigns that end in tears as she finds herself surrounded by the contents of emptied cupboards and forgotten drawers, too exhausted to do anything but despair at the mess she has created.

These typical experiences from each trimester can be helpfully understood in yoga terms as expressions of changes to the energy body or 'pranamaya kosha'. In the same way as the asanas in the previous chapter help to develop strength and mobility in the physical body, freeing it from the effects of injury and strain, so too practices which work directly with pranamaya kosha can help to manage exhaustion and erratic energy throughout pregnancy by improving and sustaining an even flow of energy.

Case study – Anna

Prior to becoming pregnant I had hardly done any yoga at all but when I started it I found that it really helped to make me feel more energized in later pregnancy. At times I felt quite exhausted but it helped me to relax and recharge my batteries.

Yoga, pregnancy and the respiratory system

Work on vitality levels begins with refining awareness of how energy moves through the body. The first place to start is with the flow of breath.

All yoga practices that work directly with the energy body have their basis in breath awareness. The air we breathe is not prana, but it contains prana, as do food, water, thoughts and emotions. Prana does not only enter the body through the breath, but breath is a major source of energy, and so the way that you breathe provides you with the most useful tool for managing levels of prana in your body. During pregnancy especially, making changes to the rhythm, depth and pace of breath is an effective way to manage vitality, particularly because there are so many challenges and changes to the respiratory system at this time.

For example, because of changes to blood composition and volume, resting breath rate and depth increase. As the baby grows and takes up more space, the diaphragm cannot move easily, and more ribcage breathing is needed. There is also increased blood flow in the nasal lining which can cause a 'stuffy' nose. The combined effect of these changes is that many pregnant women experience breathlessness on exertion, so it is important to learn to pace yourself, taking appropriate rest and managing changing breath patterns.

Breath and movement synchronization for management of energy

In Chapter 02, you were introduced to the basic forms of four core breaths. In the previous chapter, you learnt how to synchronize breath and movement in order to strengthen and mobilize the physical body. In the following practices, further developments of the core breaths are followed by a series of physical movements that are simpler and more rhythmic than those in the previous chapter, so you may direct more attention to conscious use of breath and develop a refined awareness of energy patterns. Wherever the mind goes, energy flows. But the mind is easily distracted. So in yoga, the sound and feel of the breath is used as a way to help the mind direct energy flows. By focusing attention on your breath patterns, you can bring a movement of mental awareness through the body, enhancing and improving the flow of energy. This chapter teaches how to develop the breath practices you have already learnt, and gives guidance on how to use these breath patterns together with rhythmic movements to free energy and boost vitality. These rhythmic movements are both visible and invisible: the first two sections (PMA and shakti bandhas) are visible bodily movements, whilst the third section (pelvic floor and inner power) directs the attention within, to the movements of the pelvic floor muscles, a vital source of strength and vitality, especially during pregnancy.

Development from the four core breaths

All these breaths require basic familiarity with the breaths in Chapter 02.

Invocation of Energy/Cosmic recharge (prana mudra)

This is a remarkably effective way to increase vitality, trust and confidence. Traditionally done facing the rising sun, this practice is a symbolic giving and receiving of energy, which creates a powerful sense of tranquillity and acceptance. This version simplifies the classical practice, without breath retentions, but with a voiced exhale.

1 Sit comfortably (p. 52). Close eyes. Have spine straight, and shoulders relaxed down from ears.

2 Rest right hand in lap, palm facing upward, cradling back of left hand. This is Bhairavi mudra. Establish Full yogic breath and watch its rhythm for three rounds.

3 As abdomen begins to expand on next inhalation (or if you are in late pregnancy, at start of inhalation), separate hands and move them up to navel height, palms facing belly and fingertips pointing towards each other but not touching. Hold palms a little in front of belly.

4 As breath moves up into chest and ribcage expands, continue to lift hands up to chest height.

5 Continuing inhalation right up to top of lungs, raise hands up to collarbones.

6 At height of inhalation, stretch open arms out to sides, bending elbows to bring hands level with top of head. Turn palms upwards and spread fingers wide.

7 Exhaling, slowly move palms back down, first to collarbones, then chest, then navel.

8 Complete exhalation by returning hands to lap, back of left palm cradled in palm of right. Relax in this position and breathe normally.

9 Repeat at least twice more, or until arms and breath are fully synchronized.

10 Then carry the voice on exhalation. Repeat first part of sequence, inhaling to lift hands up above head, but this time on exhalation, allow a long 'aum' sound to carry out with breath as hands lower down.

11 Repeat three more times, and return to an awareness of natural rhythm of breath as you sit with hands in Bhairavi mudra.

Tips

In late pregnancy, this is most enjoyably done sitting on a birthing ball or chair (p. 74). Give 'bump clearance' by keeping hands a little way away from body. Keep shoulders relaxed down as you raise hands. As you synchronize breath with arm motions, begin to move your mental awareness with rise and fall of breath. Inhaling, draw mental awareness from base of spine to top of head. Exhaling, let awareness descend from top of head to base of spine. At height of exhalation, when hands are open and arms wide, the physical posture creates an invitation for energy to enter the body. It is a gesture which can be practiced anywhere by recognizing every inhalation as an invitation for energy to revitalize the body.

Punctuated golden thread exhalation

This variation on Golden thread exhalation lengthens the out-breath, releasing the body deeper into a resting and healing space. Even within this pattern of consciously extended exhalation, the rhythmic breath cycle is still respected, and as much of the Full yogic breath as feels accessible is used throughout.

1 Follow instructions for Golden thread exhalation (p. 18).

2 Then simply alter the exhalation by putting little pauses along its length: exhale – pause – exhale – pause – exhale – pause. Instead of one continuous thread, there is a series of pauses along length of exhalation.

3 Divide up breath however feels easiest, exhale – pause, exhale – pause, as if the breath were a sentence, and the pauses commas. Put in as many pauses as feels comfortable along length of breath. This further extends exhalation, and deepens power of out-breath as an antidote to pain and tension.

Spiral thread exhalation with punctuation

1 Follow instructions for Punctuated golden thread exhalation above.

2 Visualize exhalation passing out in the shape of a corkscrew, spiralling round after every pause. Start with just one spiral, and then extend the number of spirals as you increase the number of pauses along the length of breath.

3 Exhale around every loop of corkscrew, and pause before breathing round next loop in the descending spiral: exhale round loop and pause, exhale round loop and pause.

4 Perhaps each loop gets smaller until you reach end of corkscrew.

5 Keep breath coming in through nose and out through mouth.

Tips

See which image works best for your length of breath: the long straight line, or the corkscrew. Choose the version that fits your length of breath. This breath can be particularly helpful during labour.

If you have trouble sleeping during pregnancy, these can be helpful breaths to help you wind down and rest well. For this it works best if you keep your mind focused by counting each breath. If you count down, for example from 11 to zero, it can feel as if each breath lowers you deeper into rest. If you are still awake, then count back up to a higher number, and then count down again. If still awake then roll over and repeat the process lying on other side. Occupying the mind by linking its focus to the breath in this way can help you to enter a restful state even if you are not fully asleep. Used in this way, the Golden thread exhalation can be very soporific. You may even find that it helps you drop off to sleep in early first stage labour, between contractions.

Ujjayi/Golden thread combination breath

As the title suggests, this practice brings together the second two core breaths described in Chapter 02. It's a combination that can arise spontaneously. Before attempting to learn this practice as a conscious activity, however, it is important to feel completely familiar with its component parts.

1 Begin with rhythmic Ujjayi breath (p. 16).
2 Wait for an exhalation and open lips slightly, allowing breath to travel out through the small gap between upper and lower lips.
3 Feel a fine cool breeze passing out between lips. Have cheeks, lips and face relaxed.
4 Keep Ujjayi breath for inhalations, and continue using Golden thread exhalation. Feel breath travelling in through nose, with soft Ujjayi sound in throat, and out through mouth. Allow exhalation to lengthen each time, without pushing or forcing, but simply letting the out-breath increase in length.
5 Keep on for as long as you want. When you are ready to stop, first let go of Ujjayi on inhalation, and hear sound of incoming breath resonating more loudly in nose. Then make an audible exhalation through lips.
6 Take a yawn, and return to natural pattern of breath.

Tips

Since this can arise as a spontaneously occurring breath, it is sometimes best to play with the relationship between the two parts, watching for a comfortable place to introduce an Ujjayi inhalation when doing Golden thread, or watching for a place to comfortably exhale with Golden thread when doing Ujjayi. Respect the natural flow of breath, and be attentive to changed patterns of pace and rate that can develop with protracted use of this combination breath. Both Ujjayi and the Golden thread reduce breath rate, so watch closely to make sure you feel comfortable with this slower pace. This combined practice is a powerful antidote to fear, panic, anxiety and any kind of stress.

Yoga remedies for erratic energy patterns

The above variations of the four core breaths lead to heightened awareness of breath patterns. It is this awareness that can gradually slow, lengthen and deepen each breath, and it is these changes which can improve vitality and help you deal with exhaustion. Because a balanced and even breath flow is calming as well as energizing, these patterns of breathing are also useful techniques for quietening the mind and promoting restful sleep.

Case study – Gloria

Gloria was having trouble sleeping. She was 24 weeks pregnant with her first baby, every night she tossed and turned, physically uncomfortable and energetically and emotionally unable to settle. Explaining her difficulties to her yoga teacher, it was suggested that she use a combined approach of supportive postures and breath and awareness practices to help her cope. In her yoga class, she practised lateral lying with support (p. 34) with a view to using this pose as her first posture in bed at night. Then she established a rhythmic Circle of breath (p. 11) and the Golden thread/Ujayii combination breath (p. 118), visualizing the exhalation travelling far way in a spiral (p. 117). During the yoga nidra practice in class, she fell into a deep sleep, so her teacher suggested that if she did find herself awake in the night, she might find it helpful not to try to return to sleep, but instead to listen to a yoga nidra relaxation practice (p. 166 and CD track 5).

The following week Gloria returned to the class smiling and fully rested: 'The change in posture and breath helped me to get to sleep much easier' she said, '…and not trying to get back to sleep in the night really took the pressure off. I just relaxed and listened to the CD, and without noticing it, found myself back asleep again. If I didn't, then I wasn't worried, because I knew I was relaxing well.'

Energy freeing series (pawanmuktasana or PMA)

This remarkable sequence combines two approaches to PMA: its basis is the series first taught by Paramahamsa Satyananda, founder of the Bihar School of Yoga (p. 233) and it includes refinements and improvements developed by Mukunda Stiles, originator of Structural Yoga Therapy (p. 233).

The sequence can be done as a whole, working through each movement in turn to energize the entire body, or you can focus on a specific area. For example, if your neck and shoulders are stiff, work with the practices for that part of the body (pp. 128–33). At a physical level, these practices can be used as effective remedies for localized aches and pains.

Case study – Claire

My shoulders became crunchy from sleeping on my left side for the benefit of the baby; so the tactics (joint freeing series pp. 128–133) I learned for opening the space between my shoulders were invaluable: when I had done them I could move my head and neck again, which was great.

Each practice usually involves a pair of movements synchronized with breath. The actions bring every joint of the body through its full range of motion, whilst the breath synchronization focuses the mind and releases blocked energy. The breath synchronization and mental focus are just as important as the movements, so before beginning each practice, establish an easy rhythm of full breath. Choose whichever of the core breaths (pp. 11–19) or variations you prefer, and repeat each pair of movements up to seven times in time with the breath.

To improve accessibility during pregnancy, the movements are grouped around the modified base positions described in Chapter 03. A recommended base position is suggested for each group, but if an alternative pose feels more comfortable (for example if you prefer to work from a chair), then do what suits you best.

From stick pose (p. 53):

Toe stretching/curling

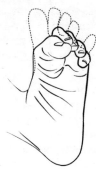

figure 4.2 Toe stretching and curling

- Inhale, spread toes as wide apart from each other as possible, pushing into heels.
- Exhale, curl toes under and squeeze.

Ankle stretching/bending

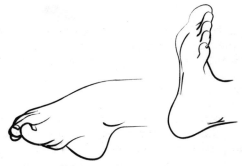

figure 4.3 Ankle stretching and bending

- Inhale, push into heels and draw toes back towards head.
- Exhale, point toes away and stretch fronts of feet.

Ankle eversion/inversion

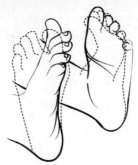

figure 4.4 Ankle eversion and inversion

- Keep heels pushed away and feet upright.
- Inhale, draw outsides of feet towards each other, bring inner arches closer together and stretch outsides of ankles.
- Exhale, push inner arches of feet away and draw outsides of feet back towards head, feel strength along outsides of legs.

Ankle rotation

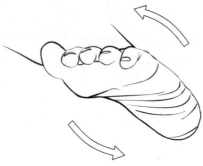

figure 4.5 Ankle rotation

- One round of breath (inhale and exhale) completes one complete circle.
- Inhale, draw semi-circle with toes and feet moving towards head, heels pushing away.
- Exhale, draw semi-circle with toes and feet moving away from head, toes pointing down.
- After seven rounds, repeat in opposite direction.

Knee flexion/extension

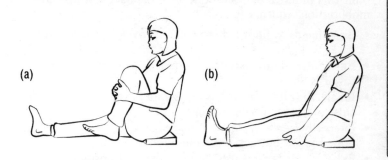

figure 4.6 a, b Knee flexion and extension

- Exhale, hold thigh close to knee with both hands from beneath and draw heel towards buttock, moving thigh towards side of belly.
- Inhale, continue to hold leg as knee straightens and push into heel.
- After seven rounds swap sides.

Hip external/internal rotation

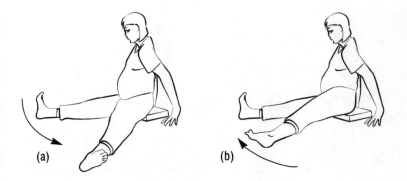

figure 4.7 a, b Hip external and internal rotation

Cautions

If you are experiencing discomfort in the pelvic joints, either omit this practice or precede it with the Sacral stabilization/mobilization sequence (p. 64).

- Bring hands to floor behind you to provide support and lean back.
- Externally rotate left leg so outside edge of foot moves towards floor.
- Inhale, slide leg outward, keeping foot flexed, with outer edge close to floor and knee straight.
- Internally rotate left leg so inside edge of foot moves towards floor and left buttock lifts from floor.
- Exhale, slide leg inwards, back to the start position, keeping foot flexed, with inner edge close to floor and knee straight.
- Repeat up to seven rounds on left and then swap sides.

Tip

To build strength and stability in this range of movement, fully engage buttock muscles.

From Cat pose (p. 39):

Incorporate seven rounds of Cat (p. 39) and Tiger (p. 47) at this point in the series before moving on to the following movements.

Hip adduction/abduction

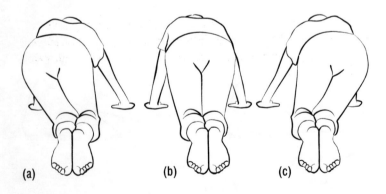

(a)　　　　　(b)　　　　　(c)

figure 4.8 a, b, c Hip adduction and abduction

- Squeeze knees and thighs together throughout this practice.
- Inhale, lower hips to right side, keeping buttocks in line with knees.
- Exhale, raise hips back to start position.
- Repeat on left side.
- Alternate between left and right sides for seven rounds.

From supported Thunderbolt/Hero seat (p. 59):

Caution

Have sufficient height beneath you so that you can maintain a comfortable seated position that brings minimal weight on to lower legs and ankles.

Hand stretches/clenches

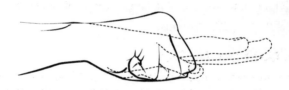

figure 4.9 Hand stretches and clenches

- Maintain arms at shoulder height and width throughout.
- Inhale, spread fingers and thumbs as wide apart as possible.
- Exhale, tuck thumb in and clench fingers around it, squeezing tight.

Wrist bends

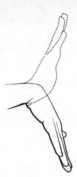

figure 4.10 Wrist bends up and down

- Maintain arms at shoulder height and width throughout.
- Inhale, push into heel of hands and point fingers and thumbs upwards.
- Exhale, point fingers and thumbs downwards.
- Repeat up to seven rounds.

Wrist side bends

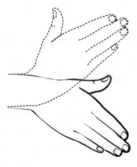

figure 4.11 Wrist side bends in and out

- Maintain arms at shoulder height and width throughout, palms facing up, fingers straight.
- Inhale, draw outer edges of hands (little finger sides) towards outer edges of forearms.
- Exhale, draw inner edges of hands (thumb sides) towards inner edges of forearms.

Wrist rotations

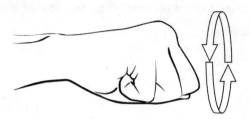

figure 4.12 Wrist rotation

- Maintain arms at shoulder height and width throughout, thumbs tucked in and fingers curled around thumbs.
- One round of breath (inhale and exhale) completes one complete circle.
- Inhale, move fists in semi circle downwards and outwards.
- Exhale, move fists in semi circle upwards and inwards.
- After seven rounds, repeat in opposite direction.

Elbow bends

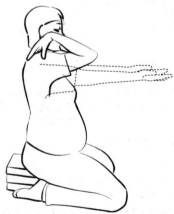

figure 4.13 Elbow bends in and out

- Maintain elbows at shoulder height and width throughout.
- Inhale, straighten elbows to bring hands to shoulder height, palms up.
- Exhale, bend elbows to bring fingertips to shoulder tops.

Elbow circling

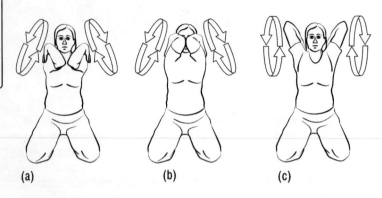

figure 4.14 a, b, c Elbow circles

- Maintain elbows bent with fingertips lightly resting on shoulder tops throughout.
- One round of breath (inhale and exhale) completes one complete circle.
- Inhale, bring elbows together in front of chest and lift as high as possible.
- Exhale, as elbows lower bring them wide out to sides and then as close together behind back as possible.

Shoulder external/internal rotation

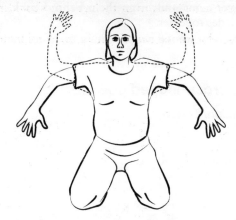

figure 4.15 Shoulder rotation external and internal

- Maintain elbows wide out to sides at shoulder height throughout.
- Inhale and bring forearms vertical with hands (palms facing forward) above elbows, at right angles to upper arms.
- Exhale, lower hands, keeping forearms vertical at right angles to upper arms.

Shoulder extension/flexion

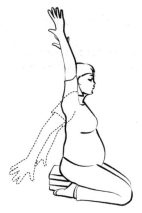

figure 4.16 Shoulder extension and flexion

- Keep arms straight at shoulder width throughout.
- Inhale, lower arms and bring them behind back, drawing shoulder blades together.
- Exhale, lift arms above head, aiming to bring them in line with ears.

From easy cross-legged pose (p. 62):

Spinal extension/flexion

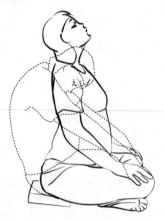

figure 4.17 Spine flexion and extension

- Rest hands on knees.
- Inhale, lifting breastbone and head, move spine forward.
- Exhale, tuck in chin and tailbone, round spine.

Spinal side bends

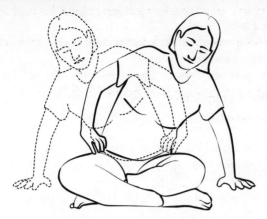

figure 4.18 Spinal side bends to the left and right

- Place right hand on right hip and left hand on floor at left side.
- Inhale, sit tall.
- Exhale bend to right side, keeping chest open and right hand on the floor.
- Swap hands and repeat on left side.
- Alternate between sides to repeat seven rounds.

Spinal rotation

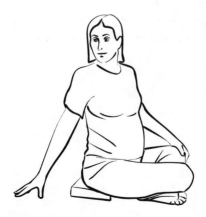

figure 4.19 Spinal rotation

- Place left hand on left knee and right hand on floor at right side.
- Inhale, sit tall.
- Exhale, twist to right side, keeping chest open.
- Inhale, return to start position.
- Alternate between sides to repeat seven rounds.

Neck flexion/extension

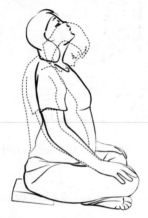

figure 4.20 Neck flexion and extension

- Inhale, sit tall, lift chin and lengthen neck.
- Exhale, drop chin to chest.

Neck side bends

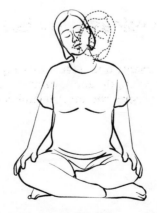

figure 4.21 Neck side bends left and right

- Inhale sit tall, lengthen neck.
- Exhale, bend neck, lowering right ear towards right shoulder whilst keeping face forwards.
- Inhale return to central position.
- Alternate on each side to repeat seven rounds.

Neck rotation

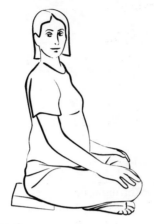

figure 4.22 Neck rotation

- Inhale sit tall, lengthen neck.
- Exhale, turn head to right, keeping chin level.
- Inhale return to central position.
- Alternate on each side to repeat seven rounds.

Energy block release practices (shakti bandhas)

These rhythmic movements free stagnant energy from the core of the body, build strength and promote mobility. Their repetitive patterns energize the mother and soothe the baby within.

Pulling the rope

From Stick pose (p. 53)

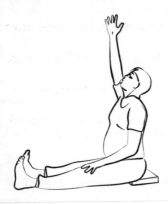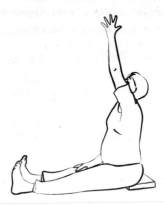

figure 4.23 Pulling the rope

- Keep arms straight throughout.
- Inhale reach right arm forward and straight up, clenching fist as if grabbing a rope.
- Exhale, draw right arm down strongly.
- Alternate on both sides to repeat seven rounds.

Churning the mill (chakki chalanasana)

From Stick pose (p. 53)

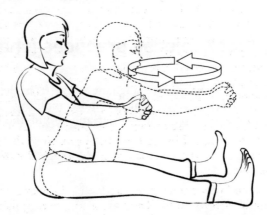

figure 4.24 Churning the mill

- Inhale, raise both arms to shoulder height.
- Exhale, interlock fingers starting with left thumb on top, and drop shoulders.
- Inhale, sit tall, bend elbows slightly.
- Exhale, tilt pelvis forward, inclining whole spine and arms forward and to right.
- Exhale, tilt pelvis backwards, inclining whole spine and arms left, back to vertical.
- One round of breath (inhale and exhale) completes one complete pelvic circle.
- Repeat seven rounds clockwise, pause, change hand interlock (bring right thumb on top) and repeat anti-clockwise.

Breath and inner power – pelvic floor pranayama

In yogic anatomy of the energy body, the muscles of the pelvic floor are considered to be the 'root': the source of power and vitality. Great significance is attached to the healthy tone and conscious control of these muscles, and there are many yoga practices incorporating perineal 'locks' (bandha) and 'seals' (mudra), which involve a contraction of pelvic floor muscles. During pregnancy, these muscles come under additional strain from supporting the weight of the contents of the womb, including the placenta, the amniotic fluids and the growing baby, so strengthening practices become especially necessary.

But strength and tone in the pelvic floor is only helpful in terms of preparing for birth if you can also learn to release these muscles. During pregnancy and birth, the capacity to release the pelvic muscles is equally important as their tone. Both depend upon an acute awareness of the actions of the muscles in the area. The system described below adapts classic yoga mudra and bandha to promote equality of tone and release in the pelvic floor. Although these practices are drawn from traditional yoga techniques, they differ in key respects from usual yoga methods. For full details of these distinctions, yoga practitioners, teachers and others with a special interest in this approach to the pelvic floor are referred to the discussions in *Mother's Breath* (see Taking it further).

These breath and pelvic floor practices are vital preliminaries to the Birthing breath (p. 206). They are also a prerequisite for effective use of the post-natal Healing breath (p. 216). Because the Birthing and Healing breaths both use synchronized breath and pelvic floor movements, it is necessary to feel which part of the pelvic floor goes where before starting to move it or trying to connect that movement with breath patterns. It is vital to know where everything is before you start. For that reason, the practices below are presented in a sequence that encourages coherent exploration of the pelvic floor. The techniques are best practised initially in the order presented below, but once you are familiar with them then you can practise them individually, and in any order.

Cautions

This form of pelvic floor awareness is suitable in pregnancy, but not for the post-natal period. For post-natal recovery, please see the Healing breath (p. 216).

Locating the pelvic floor

For this exploration of the different parts of the pelvic floor, it is best to take downward pressure of weight off the pelvic floor by resting forwards, with knees in a wide kneeling position and sufficient soft support under the head to feel comfortable. There is no need to bring the head right down to the floor, and certainly avoid doing this if it makes you feel nauseous or uncomfortable. Instead, have head level with hips or higher, for example as in supported Hare pose (p. 40). If kneeling forward is uncomfortable then sitting astride a bolster and tilting forwards can work well, but is best done with support (p. 61).

Although these forward tilting options have the advantage of taking weight off the pelvic floor, they may not be comfortable enough for you to really focus attention on the pelvic floor sufficiently to understand what is happening. In these cases (for example if you experience heartburn or dizziness when you rest forwards), then it is better to practise from an upright position, with the knees wide, either sitting on a chair or a bolster. Alternatively, sitting on a large exercise/birthing ball provides the opportunity to roll your weight forwards and backwards to better direct attention into the various areas of the pelvic floor.

Guidance for all pelvic floor practices

1 Settle posture comfortably, choose the core breath with which you feel most at ease, and breathe at a pace that allows for

lifts, squeezes and releases to flow gently, synchronized with breath.

2 Go at your own pace; feel comfortable and relaxed with the rhythm of the breath as it paces your explorations of the pelvic floor. It is best to do these practices with eyes closed.

3 Establish a movement of awareness up and down the spine in time with breath.

4 Inhaling, move mental attention from base of spine to crown of head and, exhaling, allow awareness to return to starting point.

5 Let synchronized rhythm of breath and awareness continue for a few cycles until it feels natural.

6 Exhaling, bring mental awareness down to base of spine, and follow instructions below for each individual practice.

7 Be sure that during each practice it is only the pelvic muscles that move. Everything else should be relaxed and still, especially face, abdomen and buttocks. Just the pelvic floor muscles are squeezing or lifting and releasing, moving at the breath's comfortable rhythm.

8 Always return to this preparation before moving to the next practice.

9 In between each practice, if you are still at ease in your original position then stay where you are, but if you need to move, make adjustments to ensure continued comfort.

Sahajoli mudra – spontaneous psychic gesture or clitoral tickle

1 This first stage draws energy right to the very front of the pelvic floor. It works muscles quite close to the pubic bone, so to start, direct attention to this bone.

2 Exhaling, let mental attention move forward to the pubic bone, right at the very front of the pelvic floor. (If you are sitting upright with support beneath you, tilt slightly forwards until you can feel some pressure coming towards the front of the pelvic floor).

3 Inhaling with awareness here, squeeze tight those muscles that would stop an imaginary flow of urine. Imagine that by squeezing tight these muscles you have completely stopped this imaginary flow.

4 Exhaling, release these muscles. Sense how this release would allow the imaginary flow of urine to resume its flow.

5 Continue for a few more rounds of easy rhythmic breath, keeping awareness at front of pelvic floor and squeezing muscles there on inhale, and releasing them on exhale. As you squeeze and release these muscles, you may feel a ticklish sensation as the hood of the clitoris is moved by the referred action of the squeeze on the urethra.

Ashwini mudra – horse gesture or anal squeeze

1 Exhaling, bring awareness down to the base of the spine, let it rest there, right at the very back of the pelvic floor. (If you are sitting upright with support beneath you, or on a ball, then tilt or roll slightly backwards until you can feel some pressure coming towards the back of the pelvic floor.)
2 Inhaling with awareness right at back of pelvic floor, squeeze tight the muscles around the anus.
3 Once you can feel this ring of muscle closing, exhale and release.
4 Continue for a few more rounds of rhythmic breath, keeping awareness at the very back of the pelvic floor, squeezing muscles there on inhale, and releasing on exhale.

Pause for pelvic geography awareness

So now be aware of the two areas you have been moving. Know that the squeezes and releases of Sahajoli and Ashwini mark out the very front and back of the pelvic floor. These two practices help you to locate the full spread of the pelvic floor, from right at the front to right at the back. The very front was where you practised the first technique (Sahajoli), and the very back is where you practised the second technique (Ashwini). If you have support beneath, you can roll forwards to the Sahajoli place – right at the front of the pelvic floor – take one squeeze and release there, and then roll right back to the anus again, taking another squeeze and release there. Be aware of the distance between the front and the back of the pelvic floor, the two places you have just been exploring, so you can rock forwards and back, from one to the other, or simply alternate the front squeeze and the back squeeze. Know that for the birth of your baby, the place that is really important to put energy, breath and focus is right in the middle of the pelvic floor, in between these two places.

Pregnancy Mula bandha – root lock or big lift

1 Exhaling, bring mental awareness down to the base of the spine and move it forwards until it comes to rest at the middle of the pelvic floor.

2 The area for focus in mula bandha is right in the centre of the pelvic floor, neither at the front, nor at the back, but in the middle. It is in between the two places you have just been squeezing, midway between the Sahajoli place at the front and the Ashwini place at the back. (If you are sitting with support beneath you, or on a ball, then tilt or roll slightly forwards and then backwards until you feel a sense of the middle place between front and back).

3 Inhaling with awareness at this central point, draw walls of the vagina in and up.

4 Feel first outer and then deep layers of muscles moving in and up: so there is more of a lift than a squeeze at the end of the inhale.

5 Follow breath to lift up as high as feels comfortable, and then, exhaling, release lift, and let go, down into the support of whatever you are sitting on.

6 Following the easy rhythm of natural breath, let this lifting and lowering movement continue: breathing in, moving up, and breathing out, lowering down.

7 Continue for a few more cycles of rhythmic breath, keeping awareness at the very centre of the pelvic floor and squeezing and lifting muscles here on inhale, and releasing them on exhale.

Tips

The instructions above integrate movement of awareness, rhythm of breath and pelvic muscle action. Initially this may seem like a lot to handle all at once, so you may find it easier just to practise the movements of the pelvic floor until you can find your way around. When you feel ready to integrate breath and awareness with pelvic floor movements, just move awareness up and down with breath at the start, and then concentrate on the muscular movements of the pelvic floor locations. As these movements become more familiar, then re-introduce the movement of awareness with breath to synchronize with the pelvic floor movements. The layers of practice are mutually supportive.

Changing hormonal levels during pregnancy can have noticeable effects on muscle tone, and the degree of pelvic floor awareness or control can vary quite a lot from one day to the next. You may discover for instance, that Mula bandha does not feel as if just one part of the pelvic floor is lifting, but as if everything is all coming up together, or it may be difficult to distinguish one area clearly from another. What matters is that you have a clear recognition of exactly what you are feeling today, and that you accept and acknowledge that feeling and then work to synchronize whatever movement is accessible to you with your breath. With practice and attention, pelvic muscle movements may be refined to a high degree, and certainly your knowledge of this area will deepen. It is best to see these practices as a way to explore and develop your understanding of the pelvic floor, and to work gently, patiently and with acceptance at whatever level of knowledge and/or movement you have right now.

Use these practices throughout pregnancy to prepare for the Birthing breath (p. 206). There is no need to do lots. The practice is more about acquiring awareness and familiarity than about doing thousands of repetitions. It is better to be modest and persistent, for example to do batches of five or ten whenever you remember, rather then to be over-ambitious, and do so many rounds that you get bored and avoid the whole practice for weeks. Little and often is the wisest approach. In order for it not to turn into a mechanical chore, always involve a holistic awareness of breath, rhythm and energy. These practices are energizing, so avoid doing them at a time when you need to sleep.

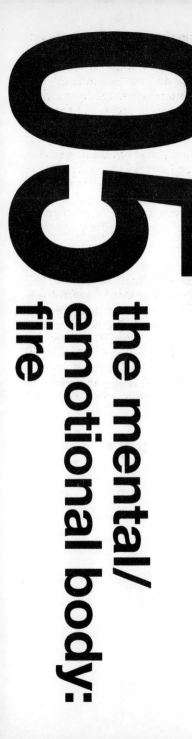

05

the mental/emotional body: fire

In this chapter you will learn:
- how yoga helps the shifting states of mind and heart in pregnancy
- yoga breath and sound practices to promote a positive bond with your unborn child
- meditation and relaxation practices to revive and restore.

Sun/Fire gesture (surya mudra)

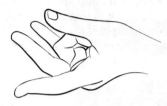

figure 5.1 Sun gesture

With hands resting palms up, comfortably on knees or thighs, lightly touch tip of ring finger to tip of thumb. Then slide ring finger to base of thumb, bending it over until fingertip is in contact with thumb pad, and thumb holding it in place, pressing on second knuckle of ring finger. The other fingers are relaxed. This hand gesture connects to the heating energy of the fire element, building qualities of expansion and digestion or consumption. In terms of the mental and emotional body, these qualities relate to the ability to handle feelings, thoughts and situations with equanimity.

Heart gesture (hridaya mudra)

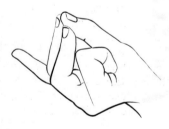

figure 5.2 Heart gesture

With hands resting palms up, comfortably on knees or thighs, lightly touch tip of index finger to tip of thumb. Then slide tip of index finger down length of thumb, bending it until fingertip is tucked into root of thumb. Keep it in this position, and touch tip of thumb to both tips of middle and ring fingers together. Little finger remains relaxed, or outstretched, whichever feels most comfortable. Traditionally this mudra is held with palms up, but if it feels easier, turn them over. This hand gesture connects to the space of the heart, enhancing qualities of compassion, love and understanding.

Both of these hand gestures can be used together with the core breaths, postures and energy practices in the previous three chapters, or with the attitudes, sound work and meditations in this chapter. They are also useful when you feel overwhelmed by unstable emotions, or proliferating worries during pregnancy.

Yoga perspectives on the mind and emotions

The aim of yoga practice is to still the mind. This stilling is ultimately in order to experience that state of 'union', of oneness which is the source of yoga, but in practical day to day terms it is a way at least to dis-identify from the endless chatter of thoughts, worries, projections and remembrances that rattle through our heads and hearts. It helps us to know that we are not our anger, or our grief, or our paranoia. Seeing the changing inner landscape of mental process for what it is, we can learn to recognize that, however disturbing they may be, our feelings pass, and we can watch them go.

During pregnancy, the tendency to identify with emotions and thoughts can increase, because there is so much more to worry about, and so many more new thoughts, experiences and concerns. It is as if the mental landscape of conscious thoughts, subconscious dreams and desires becomes more vivid. Certainly there is as much psychological work to be done during pregnancy as there are physical adaptations to be made. So yoga practices directed at the mind can be of great comfort and practical use.

Psychological work of pregnancy

Some of the changes affecting the nervous system at a physical level can also impact directly upon mental and emotional life. For example, hormone-induced changes which affect joints and the functioning of digestive, respiratory and circulatory systems can also prompt mood swings, anxiety and sleep problems. It is common in pregnancy to experience some memory loss and to notice an inability to concentrate. Increased fluid in tissues can also compress some nerves, for example causing carpal tunnel syndrome.

So in both physical and psychological terms, maternal adaptations to pregnancy are characterized by *softening* and *opening*: at a physical level this affects movement, posture and bodily rhythms, but at a mental and emotional level it can include tearfulness, disturbing or vivid dreams, acute anxiety, fear, and volatile shifts between periods of depression and elation. Much of this psychological work is necessary preparation for motherhood: fears and anxieties, for example, can help you to work through worst case scenarios concerning the health of your unborn child; disturbing dreams or tearfulness can ventilate long buried emotions about your own childhood, or provide the impetus to resolve difficult relationships that may limit your ability to transform yourself from a daughter into the kind of mother you would like to be.

Using the core breaths to calm the mind and emotions

The primary breaths promote emotional stability and adaptability. This is useful when managing the psychological work of pregnancy. For example, after experiencing the shock that comes from the simplest or most alarming physical or psychological disruption, use Ujjayi (p. 16) to centre yourself again. Notice your level of alarm, and then just take four or five breaths in Ujjayi again, as if it were drawing you back to your inner world of quiet and peace. Let the sound of the breath get louder if you like, so that it sounds louder than the thoughts in your head, or reminds you of the waves of the ocean crashing on the shore of your favourite beach, real or imaginary. This is the fast track to a relaxed breath and quieter state of mind. Any of the core breaths work well for this purpose, but to be effective, it is necessary to be familiar enough with your chosen breath for it to become second nature, and thus immediately accessible at moments of crisis or emotional challenge.

There is an intimate connection between energy levels and emotional experience. For example, volatile mood swings may be especially difficult to handle if you are feeling tired, but can become more manageable after a period of rest or settled breath. For this reason, many of the practices described in the previous chapter on the energy body are also useful in managing the unpredictable emotional and mental life of pregnancy. If you feel that low vitality or exhaustion is exacerbating the difficulties of mood swings or memory loss, then precede the practices in this chapter by a round or two of the Invocation of energy (p. 115) or two or three moves from the Energy freeing series (p. 120).

Heart/womb breath

The concept of the heart-womb connection exists both in Ayurveda, the Indian medical system closely allied with yoga, and in traditional Chinese medicine. It is an energetic link between the mother's heart and her womb. It is said to open during pregnancy, to enable the mother to nourish the child in the womb with the emotional energy of her loving heart. This special connection is the basis for this very calming and nurturing breath and awareness practice.

1 Sit in a comfortable and sustainable position with eyes closed. Breathe fully.

2 Place left palm on chest over heart and place right palm over womb, resting hand on belly, at whatever height seems to provide a strong connection with your unborn child.

3 Exhaling, settle focus of attention into womb, feeling warmth where right palm rests on belly.

4 Inhaling, move mental awareness from belly up to heart, feeling warmth where left palm rests on chest.

5 Exhaling, send mental awareness back down from heart to womb.

6 Continue with easy rhythm of breath, moving awareness from womb (right palm) to heart (left palm) with each inhalation, and sending awareness from heart to womb with each exhalation.

7 Sit breathing with this awareness for as long as you feel comfortable (maybe, with practice, up to 20 minutes).

8 When you are ready, remove hands from belly and heart, and bring palms together at chest. Breathe three more rounds and then open eyes.

Tips

This is an especially helpful breath to use when you want to restore or create a deeper connection to the presence of your unborn child, for example if you have had a particularly busy time and have almost forgotten that you are pregnant. It can feel a natural step to develop the breath and awareness practice described above into a complete meditation (p. 163).

Voicing feelings through sounded breaths

Very often, a yoga class is a silent place and yoga practice is a silent time. The only sounds heard are instructions given by the teacher, and the rhythmic breathing of the students. Whilst this silence can be a comfort and a respite from the usually noise-polluted world we inhabit, to practise only in silence is to miss a whole dimension of yoga practice that can be of great practical benefit in the management of emotions and thoughts. Pre-natally, all manner of sounds (formal and informal, conscious and spontaneous) can be used to extend the exhalation, to create sonic massage for babies, and to free breath and voice for pain management during labour. The sounds described below range from naturally occurring yawns and sighs to bija (seed) mantras. Almost any form of voice or sound work can become a natural and helpful companion to yoga breath and movement, both during pregnancy and in post-natal recovery (p. 218).

Using sound in your yoga practice during pregnancy benefits not only you, but your baby too.

Case study – Donna

Having done mostly silent yoga practice on her first pregnancy, Donna explains how many of the practices in this chapter were especially helpful to her: 'Throughout this pregnancy I have done a lot more chanting/sounded pranayama practices than I did last time – bhramari (p. 151) and variations, and chakra shuddhi (sonic massage, p. 148). I have found these very soothing, balancing, and energizing and my baby seems to love them too. Through the yoga humming and sound practices, I feel I have really discovered more about the depth of how they help me connect on a deeper level both with my baby and with my own mood changes – allowing them to be, and then (hopefully!) to pass. I have also really enjoyed the stillness that comes after the soundings.'

Sometimes it is very uncomfortable to begin to make sounds. There are frequently all sorts of shyness and obstacles towards using a voice for anything other than talking. If you begin by making the kind of sounds that come fairly naturally, like yawning and sighing and saying your own name, then you can 'sneak up' on the other sound practices, such as mantras, and find that you actually enjoy them. After all, the sound you make is simply another form of exhalation, your voice carried out into the world by the out-breath. In the techniques described below, 'Natural soundings to release' come before more formal practices with mantras, and this order of practice is the most accessible, especially if you have done no previous voice work.

Natural soundings to release

The easiest way explore these sounds is to do them in Cat (p. 39), eyes closed.

1 Begin by observing the natural breath. Breathe in and out through nose.
2 Open jaw and release it by wiggling it from side to side. Take a series of yawns. Start with small ones, and let them get bigger and louder. Four or five is good, although often when you get started it is difficult to stop. Let yawns be a vehicle to carry your voice.
3 Pause and return to natural, quiet rhythmic breath.
4 Let head hang, and allow hips to move in big easy circles, as if the circle's middle point were between the knees.
5 Relax jaw and start to sigh on each exhale. Let sighs be loud and long, repeat five or six times.
6 Circle shoulders, as if the circle's middle point were between the thumbs.
7 Take a break, resting forwards in Hare pose (p. 40).
8 Return for a few rounds to rhythmic natural breath.
9 Come back into Cat. Either return to the circles you were making before, or make a figure of eight shape connecting shoulder circles with hip circles, a free form movement with which the body is comfortable.
10 As movement becomes rhythmical, release jaw and let exhalation be a long, slow, breathy sigh carrying the sound 'ahhh'.
11 Repeat twice more, and move on to an 'eeeh' sound for three cycles.

12 Then round lips for three 'oooh' sounds. Find the sound you (and/or your baby) seem to enjoy best, and repeat a few more rounds.

13 Finally, use these movements and open jaw to sound through the vowels in your own name, or the name of your baby. For example, a mother named Eliza, with a son called Joe may find herself sounding, 'eeeh, iiih, aaah, oooh'.

14 Repeat sounds along exhalation, slow or fast as you prefer.

Tips

The sounds do not need to be very loud. In fact at the start, it is easier to make them quietly. As you increase your comfort and familiarity with the practices though, be prepared for volume to increase. These natural soundings are a useful way to release tension and relax in pregnancy, taking downward pressure of weight off pelvic floor, and creating sonic massage for the unborn baby. They are also a helpful way to practice using sound for pain management in labour (p. 206).

Sound with movement

As a means to release difficult feelings and thoughts, the sounds described above can be helpfully incorporated into any of the Energy freeing series (p. 120) and Energy block releasing practices (p. 133). For example, if you feel a particular emotion weighing heavy on your heart, use Elbow circling (p. 128) together with 'aaah' sounds on every exhale to free the heart energy from its burden. If the endless circling of a particular thought pattern troubles you, then use Churning the mill (p. 134) with 'oooh' sounds on each exhale to take your attention beyond the vicious circle. Best of all, if there are unspoken words or buried feelings from which you wish to be free, practise the Fierce goddess pose (p. 94) with the loudest 'haaa' you can manage, sticking out your tongue as far as it will go as you drop into the squat.

Pre-natal sonic massage for babies – with bija (seed) mantras

Hearing is one of the first senses to develop. Most babies in the womb are able to hear by 15 weeks. To start with, they hear mostly the internal workings of the mother's body echoing through the amniotic fluid, but in later weeks they recognize sounds of different voices, primarily the mother's voice, which resonates to them through the water in which they float.

As well as hearing the mother's voice, the baby also experiences sound vibrations as a form of sonic massage which completely surrounds them and is detected both by the sense of hearing, and by the sense of touch. The baby actually feels the mother's voice. Any sounds will do, but the mantras given below are particularly resonant, with long 'mmmm' sounds that are equally comforting for mother and child.

In yoga, every place in the body has mantra, a seed sound that contains and expresses the energy at its location. The resonance of these sounds, and the internal focus which they bring, can be both soothing and energizing. These humming sound practices are a meditative method to heighten awareness of energy centres in the body. They also, like the Golden thread, naturally extend the exhalation. The bija mantras used in Pre-natal and Post-natal sonic massage (p. 218) have no literal meaning, but their sound is associated with the elements earth, water, fire, air and ether, or space. In the tradition of yoga tantra from which this practice is derived, these elements are located in the energy body at specific centres known as chakras, or spiralling wheels of energy. Each chakra has its own element and its own Sanskrit name, which is given after the English translation in the instructions below. For a good introductory discussion of chakras, see 'Psychic Physiology of Yoga' in *Asana, Pranayama, Mudra, Bandha*, pp. 513–24 (see Taking it further).

If you find it helpful to locate the energy centres with a physical trigger, then follow the extra instructions (in brackets) at the start of each section below.

For each energy centre:

1 Sit comfortably upright, with eyes closed.
2 Establish Full yogic breath (p. 13) or Ujjayi (p. 16).
3 Exhaling, bring mental focus to level of each chakra described below.
4 Follow directions for bija mantra at each chakra, sounding three repetitions, and resonating 'mmm'.
5 Return to three rounds of your chosen quiet breath between each energy centre.

Earth centre (muladhara chakra)

1 Bring mental focus down to base of spine. (Gentle Mula bandha (p. 139) gives a useful connection to this area.)
2 Hold mental awareness here, repeating mantra 'lam'.

Water centre (swadhisthana chakra)

1 Move awareness higher up, resting attention in centre of body at level of pubic bone. (Drawing Mula bandha higher towards cervix can be an effective way to bring focus of mental attention into pelvic bowl.)

2 Hold awareness here and move attention back towards sacrum at this level, repeating mantra 'vam'.

Fire centre (manipura chakra)

1 Move awareness higher up, resting attention in centre of body at navel level. (Gentle abdominal breath and/or resting thumbs at navel with fingers pointing down can be a vivid focus to connect to this area.)

2 Hold awareness here, breathing into belly, then move attention back to spine at this level, repeating mantra 'ram'.

Air centre (anahata chakra)

1 Move awareness higher up, resting attention in centre of body at level of shoulder blades. (A big expansion to open chest on inhale, lifting sternum, provides helpful focus for this area.)

2 Hold awareness here repeating mantra 'yam'.

Ether/space centre (vishuddhi chakra)

1 Move awareness higher up, resting attention in centre of neck at level of base of throat. (Drawing Ujayii breath right up to collarbones and feeling movement at base of throat – or even touching fingertips there – can be a clear connection with this area.)

2 Hold awareness here, repeat mantra 'ham'.

Beyond elements (sahasra chakra)

1 Move awareness higher up, resting attention in centre of head at eyebrow level. (It can be easier to connect with this centre if you lick your thumb and touch the point between the two eyebrows, feeling the cool damp spot at the 'third eye' centre.)

2 Hold awareness here, repeating mantra 'aum'.

3 At the end of last 'aum', exhale, breathing awareness back down to base of spine.

4 With slow Ujjayi, for next seven breath cycles let focus of attention flow down spine with each exhalation, from top of head to tailbone. Let inhalations take care of themselves, and focus all attention on downward movement of energy and awareness, beginning each exhalation at top of head and letting awareness flow down to reach base of spine at end of every exhalation.

5 Complete with seven Full yogic breaths and no specific focus of awareness, just resting with the easy rhythm of breath.

Tips

Focus on the 'mmm' part of the mantras, since this is the sound most clearly experienced by the baby in the womb. The resonance of the sound in your body is more important than a loud, outwardly directed voice. Each person finds awareness of these energy centres in their own way, and the locations described above may not precisely match your own experience. With practice, and sensitive awareness you can learn to refine your perception of the precise points where resonance is most clearly experienced.

You can repeat the bija mantras out loud, or hear them silently. If you are voicing sound, then you can do it slowly, with one sound lasting the length of the exhalation, or more rapidly, with repetitions for the length of the exhale. You can also alternate long and short repetitions. A shift in the pitch of the humming sounds can enhance embodied understanding of the energy centres. Settle on a note at the bottom of your voice range for the first centres, and progress upwards, raising the pitch a tone at a time. If you have time, at the end of the last 'aum', reverse the process, and chant back down to base of spine. These are powerful sounds. If you experience strong physical or emotional responses to any or all of them, it can be reassuring to speak about your experiences with a yoga teacher who has an understanding of the effects of these mantras.

This energizing and focusing practice is valuable throughout pregnancy. The sounds are calming and soothing during turbulent emotional life. It is a remarkably effective method to focus attention within the body, so it is helpful when thoughts and feelings are being drawn too much outward. The sounds of the mantras have a soothing effect upon the baby within the belly, and provide the basis for shared practice once the child is born. If you enjoy the sounds of the bija mantras you may choose to use them during childbirth.

Humming bee breath (bhramari)

A calming practice to use throughout pregnancy, bhramari is a special way to communicate directly with the growing baby. The resonance of the humming sounds create vibrations which travel through the amniotic waters to give the baby a form of sonic massage similar to the mantra chanting. In this practice, closing the ears deepens the resonance for you too.

Bhramari lowers blood pressure, and the feelings of tranquillity that it promotes make it an ideal pranayama to do before any relaxation practice. It also heightens the sense of mother and baby occupying your own interior world. This makes it a helpful early evening practice to assist in the transition from work to home. Classic yoga texts claim the most noticeable effect of this breath is to induce a feeling of happiness. It certainly makes most mothers smile as they do it. Because of its tendency to promote feelings of contentment and well-being, bhramari is a useful tool during those times in pregnancy when your emotions feel volatile or unsettled.

1 Sit comfortably, eyes closed, and establish a complete yogic breath (p. 15).
2 Inhaling, raise arms, drawing elbows out wide at shoulder height.
3 Block ears (with heels of hand, index fingers or thumbs, whichever you prefer).
4 Exhaling, resonate a humming sound. It is felt more than heard, so don't strain to make it loud.
5 Focus awareness of sound vibrations in centre of chest.
6 Allow for sound to fade at end of exhalation, then start again.
7 Either keep hands in position throughout however many rounds you choose to do (seven or eleven is good to start), or raise and lower hands as necessary: for example, after every third cycle, or after every cycle if arms feel tired.

Tips

Feel that this practice is flowing freely, never strain for breath. Let it flow. If the natural rhythm of your breath is compromised, then pause and breathe normally for a few rounds. Focus on the sensations of the sound, for yourself and inside the belly where the baby experiences the vibrations as a sonic massage.

Protective egg

Once you are comfortable with Ujjayi (p. 16), deepen its interiorizing and tranquillizing effects with this variation. The Protective egg combines Ujjayi with movement of mental awareness, in a simple visualization that can be used as a protective breath practice, particularly when you feel the need for a psychic buffer or barrier between yourself and the outside world.

1 Establish an easy rhythm of quiet Ujjayi.
2 Inhaling, bring mental awareness up your spine, from tailbone to top of head, as if you were breathing up your back.
3 Exhaling Ujjayi, bring mental awareness down front of body, from top of head to base of pubic bone, as if you were breathing over face and belly.
4 Once exhalation is complete, shift awareness underneath body, returning to hold focus at base of spine.
5 This completes a full circuit of the oval 'egg shaped' movement of awareness. Let this movement of mental awareness continue with each breath cycle in synchronized flow.

Tips

With mental awareness moving in this way, it is as if the breath describes the shape of a giant egg around the body. Visualize yourself and your baby sheltered safely inside the protective shell of this egg. The visualization becomes especially clear if you imagine the breath as a moving point of golden light travelling around your body.

This practice is especially helpful at those moments in pregnancy when you feel anxious or troubled, particularly by the attitudes, comments or behaviour of others. If you find yourself in an environment whose atmosphere you dislike, or if you feel under threat in any way, then anxiety can be relieved by the practice of this breath, visualizing the shape of the breath's 'egg' as a protective shell around yourself and your baby.

Breath and focus (trataka)

This is a form of consciously directed gazing combined with breath awareness. As a technique for promoting clarity of focus and concentration, it is useful throughout pregnancy. It provides a stable focus for breath and mind and is a helpful prelude to meditation. When practised repeatedly it becomes quite automatic, and seems to happen by itself very easily. During first stage labour (p. 200), trataka can be a useful adjunct to the Golden thread breath.

1 Sit comfortably and establish steady Golden thread exhalation (p. 18).
2 Allow your eyes to focus on a point ahead of you, just far enough away that you can keep it in focus. If you are long or short-sighted, fix the focus at a distance you can see comfortably without glasses or contact lenses.

3 Then, as exhalation spins out between the lips, imagine the thread of breath is reaching towards the point upon which your eyes are focused, and that it just touches that point at the end of exhalation.

4 Inhaling, breathe in through the nose.

5 Exhaling, let each breath reach out in front to touch the point upon which your eyes are focused.

Tips

It can be helpful to use a special image or object for this practice; anything that holds a particular sacred or safe feeling for you can be helpful, because it is as if you breathe yourself into the heart of this image with every breath.

If the pace of breath changes, you may need to alter the rate at which the Golden thread exhalation breath travels to the object of visual focus. For example, if the breath slows down, then allow for the Golden thread to spin out more slowly, but if breath speeds up, then encourage the Golden thread to travel more rapidly towards the object of visual focus. In either case, the moment at which the Golden thread breath reaches the object of focus should be the precise time at which you reach the end of your natural exhalation.

Trataka with the gaze directed at an external object is called bahir (outer) trataka, and its sister practice, antar (inner) trataka directs the focus of attention inside. To practice 'inner' trataka, you either need to have such a clear image of the object of outer focus that you can replicate it inside your head when your eyes close, or you can summon up the image in the mind's eye without need for the actual object. Some women find that this inner focus is more helpful for them during labour, especially if the object of their focus is a place in which they feel especially safe and secure. With inner trataka, it is as if the Golden thread breath leads the focus of mental attention deep inside, to enter the mental image. You can also combine the outer and inner focuses by alternating periods of closed and open eyes.

Breath balancing (swara)

In yoga the flow of the breath in the nostrils is called swara. Day and night, the flow of breath naturally shifts from one nostril to the other, typically changing after about 90 minutes of flow. At any given point, the dominant nostril is the one through which the breath can be sensed to flow most easily. If left nostril dominates, then the right hemisphere of the brain is most active, and vice versa. This practice balances the flow of breath in right and left nostrils, which has a direct impact upon brain function. By becoming aware of natural changes in the flow of breath you can become more sensitive to the range of activities and attitudes that are most suited to whichever nostril, and thus whichever hemisphere of the brain is dominant.

The science of swara, or the study of changing flows of breath, is a fascinating branch of yoga dedicated to developing a continuous awareness of the flow of breath in the nostrils to create balance and poise at every level. Different characteristics are attributed to the flow of breath in right and left nostrils, and attempts to balance these flows, or to respond appropriately to the nature of breath flowing at any given time, promote equanimity and adaptability. These two qualities are especially valuable when managing the heavy psychological workload of pregnancy. Breath balancing is very useful in moments of panic or fear, because focus on breath flow brings an opportunity to distance ourselves from current circumstances. Also, the sensation of the arms wrapped around the front of the body, and warmth under the armpits is very comforting, like giving yourself a hug.

This practice is based upon the simple fact that any pressure brought under the armpits directly influences flow of breath in the nostrils. If pressure is applied under the right armpit, then breath in the left nostril tends to flow. If pressure is applied in the left armpit, then breath in the right nostril tends to flow.

1 Sit in any comfortable position with straight spine, and let shoulders drop away from ears.
2 With hands resting on thighs, watch breath as you establish a full yogic inhalation and exhalation.
3 Observe which nostril is dominant, by sensing which flow of breath is stronger. It can be helpful to breathe onto the back of your hand to detect which nostril has the more powerful flow of air.
4 When breath is rhythmic and even, cross arms over chest, tucking fingers of right hand under left armpit and fingers of left hand under right armpit. Thumbs are free, and rest on front of arm, pointing up towards shoulder.
5 Work fingers deep into warmth of armpits, and let elbows drop down.
6 Close eyes and focus attention on flow of breath into and out of nostrils.

7 Be aware of a triangular pattern of breath, as air flows into the two nostrils (the base of the triangle) and up sides to tip of triangle at point between two eyebrows.

8 Be aware of that same triangle as breath flows down from bridge of nose to the two nostrils.

9 Watch the balancing of breath in this triangle of the nose, and when it feels even, sit with the breath for as long as feels comfortable.

10 To come out, release hands from under armpits and rest backs of hands on thighs.

11 Observe pattern of flow of breath in nostrils. Note any changes that may have occurred.

Tips

It is the mental focus upon the balancing of breath that makes this practice most effective. If your arms get tired, just release hands down by sides. If you are tired, you can also balance the breath lying down. Bear in mind that if you lie on the right side, breath will tend to flow on the left nostril, and if you lie on the left side, breath will tend to flow in the right nostril.

You can do this practice sitting in a chair. It can be very inconspicuous, so you can experience its calming benefits when travelling by train, plane, bus, or even in a traffic jam. It promotes an even, measured pattern of breath, encourages efficient digestion, and is an effective way to centre yourself rapidly. Balancing the breath even for a couple of minutes creates a calm and attentive frame of mind.

Psychic alternate nostril breathing (anuloma viloma)

This is a hands-free version of the classic yoga alternate nostril breathing practice, nadi shodhana. Because of the tendency towards a stuffy nose during pregnancy, the hands-free variation is easier. It is an excellent method of creating balance and calm. In first trimester, when excitement and anxiety can be overwhelming, psychic alternate nostril breathing is very settling. During the sometimes volatile emotional swoops of middle trimester, it can bring focus and clarity. During the last trimester, it is a reliable route to achieving equanimity of emotional response in the lead-up to birth.

1 Sit comfortably, close eyes and breathe fully.
2 Sense flow of breath in nostrils, and imagine the shape of a triangle in the nose, so that the two nostrils form base corners of triangle and the point between the eyebrows is the top of triangle.
3 Feel inhalation moving up the two sides of the triangle to its tip, and exhalation moving down from tip to base.
4 Inhaling, direct focus of mental attention into left nostril, and follow breath up to tip of triangle.
5 Exhaling, direct focus of mental attention from tip of triangle to follow breath down right nostril and out at base of triangle.
6 Inhaling, direct focus of mental attention into base of right nostril, and follow flow of breath up to tip of triangle.
7 Exhaling, direct focus of mental attention from tip of triangle to follow breath down left nostril and out at base of triangle.
8 One complete round draws inhalation up through left nostril, exhalation out and down through right nostril, inhalation up through right nostril and exhalation out and down through left nostril.
9 Feel triangle of breath in nose, and imagine it flowing up and down each side.
10 Repeat five rounds and pause for a round of Full yogic breath with awareness in both nostrils.

Tips

Keep breath flowing in an easy rhythm, and allow awareness to move only at pace of breath. As an 'invisible' pranayama that no one else can see that you are doing, Psychic alternate nostril breathing is a handy practice to use in daily life: in crowded buses or trains, in cars, and during stressful moments at work or home. Awareness of the rhythm of triangular flow of breath can help restore balance, equanimity and poise when you are under pressure.

Entrainment breathing

This breath is for two, or more, and promotes a profound connection between those who practise it together. 'Entrainment' means a process of leading, following or matching your partner in such a way as to bring two people into rhythmic connection. This comforting, reassuring practice can relieve anxiety and promote feelings of well-being. It is profoundly reassuring and relaxing, and can be used to settle you back to sleep if you wake in the night. Throughout pregnancy it can provide you and your partner with a special way to rest together with the baby.

Sit in close contact with a friend, relative or partner. Either sit back to back (p. 58), or so that your partner has his or her back supported by the wall and their legs out wide enough so you can sit in between them, and rest your spine against their belly. The supporting partner can bend their knees if it is more comfortable. This also works well if you lie down together on your sides to make 'spoons' with your back cradled by your partner's front. This can be a more sustainable position in which to use this breath for any extended period.

1 Both close your eyes. Breathe fully.
2 After a few rounds, notice how your breathing patterns may start to fit together.
3 Observe how the partner, simply by paying close attention to the rhythm of your breath, can allow their own breath to fall into your patterns of inhalations and exhalations.
4 Allow for this cooperative rhythmic dance of the two breaths together to continue for as long as you are both comfortable.

Tips

The heart of this practice is compassionate awareness and mutual respect. As you begin to observe the breathing patterns, the two rhythms can effortlessly fall into step. With practice, you may notice that you can shorten the length of time it takes for the two distinct breathing rhythms to come together.

Sometimes it can be hard to hear your breath at first, and so a loudly audible Ujjayi (p. 16) can reduce the strain of listening. It can be useful to use this first, and then let it fade as the emphasis comes to be more on the movement of the breath than the sound.

It can be difficult for the partner to be able to follow your breath easily, and it takes some practice to get used to breathing in someone else's rhythm. Also, some partners may not be able to sustain the Entrained breath without becoming breathless and anxious themselves. In these cases it is worth dipping in and out of the Entrained breath, for example letting your partner follow your breath for as long as is comfortable, and then breathing naturally in their own rhythm for a while before returning to the Entrained breath pattern.

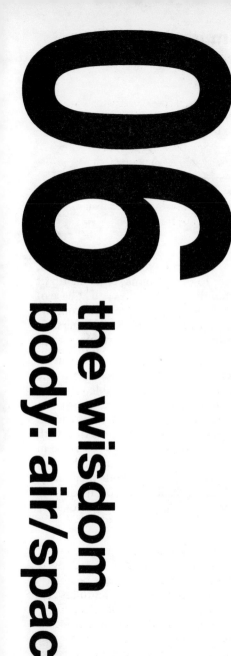

06

the wisdom body: air/space

In this chapter you will learn:
- about understanding and wisdom in preparation for motherhood
- yoga breath and sound practices to encourage insight and trust
- yoga meditations to promote calm and receptivity.

Air gesture (vayu mudra)

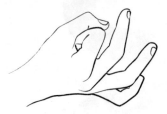

figure 6.1 Air gesture

With hands resting palms up, comfortably on knees or thighs, lightly touch tip of index finger to tip of thumb. Slide the tip of index finger down length of thumb until it reaches pad at base of thumb, where it is held in place by the gentle pressure from the thumb on the first joint of the index finger. The other fingers are relaxed or stretched out, whichever is most comfortable.

This hand gesture connects to the energy of the air element, enhancing qualities of movement and change. In relation to the yoga body of wisdom, it connects to the invisible, shifting process of the subconscious mind which provides flashes of insight and understanding beyond our ability for rational deduction or emotional response. It can be used together with the core breaths (Chapter 02), or with the practices described in Chapters 03–06. It is also a useful gesture when you feel the need for guidance, or deeper understanding during your pregnancy, for example when faced with difficult decisions or apparently irresolvable circumstances that defy your capacity for logic or heartfelt response.

Knowledge gesture (gyan mudra)

Vayu mudra is closely related to gyan mudra (psychic gesture of knowledge)

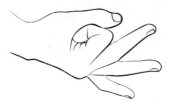

figure 6.2 Knowledge gesture

In this gesture, the position of the index finger is basically the same as for Air gesture, but is maintained by tucking tip of index finger into root of thumb, where it remains held by the gentle inward pressure from the thumb. For gyan mudra, palms face down. Gyan is a more interiorizing mudra than the widely practised chin mudra (same gesture with palms up), which creates a greater sense of receptivity and openness. It is a helpful hand gesture to accompany breath and awareness practices in this chapter because it focuses the mind inwards, enhancing access to insight which comes during higher states of consciousness.

Yoga perspectives on wisdom

Wisdom naturally occurs when an individual connects with the unity of consciousness that is the source and aim of all yoga. Insights, clear perception, and intuitive guidance all come through a quiet mind and an open heart. The practices in previous chapters are intended to create the stable physical, psychological and energetic foundations for such experiences. Calm mental focus and open-hearted acceptance leads to a place of understanding and trust from where it is natural to make wise choices and appropriate decisions. In this place, petty or selfish concerns melt away and priorities change, so that a sense of the universal 'rightness' of what is appropriate and timely becomes more important than everyday worries.

In yoga, this connection with the source of insight and universal wisdom is in the realm of 'vigyanomaya kosha': the level of being that enables humans to act neither for personal gain, nor because of subconscious desires and aversions, but because they are guided instead by the clear light shining from the essential unity of all consciousness. At certain times in a person's life, for example, during pregnancy, childbirth and whilst mothering infants, this light can seem to shine more brightly than usual. It is as if, during this time in a woman's life, her physical and energetic connection to natural patterns of growth, ripening and nurture can lead to intuitive wisdom.

Inner guidance during pregnancy

One of the most challenging, and least acknowledged, maternal adaptations to pregnancy is that a woman suddenly becomes, by simple virtue of being pregnant, a magnet for everybody's comments about pregnancy, childbirth, motherhood and baby care. Whilst pregnant, you are likely to receive much advice, not all of it welcome. Relatives, well-meaning care-givers and even strangers often see a pregnant woman as a captive audience for their own stories, experiences and opinions, or as a willing recipient of books and other materials, all pedalling their particular angle on childbirth and family life. Sometimes these pieces of advice are good information, which may be helpful, but they may be frightening, upsetting or annoying. Showered with such offerings, it can be hard to know how to respond. Yoga helps you to maintain your equanimity as you access your own inner wisdom.

All the breathing and postures (Chapters 02, 03 and 04) which boost energy and promote poise and flexibility can help to grow your confidence in the face of a flood of well-meaning comments, but it is practices which encourage mental and emotional stability (Chapter 05) and techniques which help you to access your own inner wisdom (this chapter) which are particularly valuable in this context. By awakening your awareness of intuitive guidance, and learning to honour its promptings, then you can readily judge the appropriate response to others' advice. For example, practices which foster your connection with your growing baby (p. 163) and an understanding of your own higher purpose as expressed in your sankalpa (p. 165), help you to welcome advice which resonates with your own intuition, and to discard without distress those comments which are of no relevance to you. By heightening, through meditation, your appreciation of the profound inner silence (p. 168) from which your clearest intuitions originate, you become untroubled by the often deafening cacophony of competing reactions to your pregnancy, because you know in your heart what it best for you and your baby. Practising all these techniques helps to develop acceptance and spontaneity in preparation for the challenges of childbirth and motherhood.

Heart/womb mudra and meditation

This practice follows from the Heart/womb breath and awareness practice (p. 145)

1 Follow instructions for Heart/womb breath. Close eyes.
2 When rhythm of breath and accompanying mental awareness are fully synchronized, gently tilt head slightly to left.
3 Sense that the slightly tilted head encourages focus of mental attention to shift down into heart.
4 Continue with movement of awareness from womb to heart (inhale) and from heart to womb (exhale).
5 Use exhalations to deepen focus on heart, by 'dropping' thoughts from head down into heart.
6 Sit breathing with this as long as you feel comfortable (maybe, with practice, up to 15 minutes).
7 When you want to stop, remove hands from belly and heart, return head to an upright position and bring palms together at chest.
8 Breathe three more rounds and open eyes.

Tip

If you find it uncomfortable to keep your head tilted, lessen the angle of tilt, and/or bring head upright every so often before returning to the tilted position. This is a deeply centring practice that harmonizes thoughts and feelings with a connection to the unborn child. It creates an attitude of heart and mind that is receptive to insights of higher wisdom.

Golden circle (seated)

One of the simplest ways to develop a connection with intuitive wisdom, and to promote the tendency for harmonious and appropriate response to the needs of yourself and your baby, is to integrate sound and breath awareness by synchronizing sounds with simple movements. Because voicing the exhalation tends to lengthen it, the synchronization of movement with sound usually involves slowing your movements to match the increased length of breath. This promotes a heightened awareness of the breath rhythm, a sense of comfort in the slowly moving body and a quietly receptive state of mind and heart.

1 Sit comfortably, and breathe fully.
2 Inhale, and at end of the next exhalation, bring palms together at chest.
3 Inhaling, lift hands, still with palms together, above head.
4 Exhaling, stretch fingers, and move arms out wide to sides, tracing a circle around you with hands as you lower them.
5 At end of exhale, finish with palms resting on belly, thumbs horizontal and touching at about navel height, fingers pointing down, index fingers touching to form a downward pointing triangle: yoni mudra (p. 37). Inhale and exhale here.
6 When you are ready to begin the next cycle of breath, bring palms back together on chest, inhale, exhale, and repeat sequence of movements, reaching up, out and down with inhale, and bringing hands back to belly for exhale.
7 Synchronize movements of arms and hands with rhythm of breath.
8 Then prepare to extend exhalations by voicing them.
9 With palms together on chest, exhale 'yam' (with a long 'mmm').
10 Inhaling, reach arms above head.
11 As arms spread wide and out down to sides, exhale 'aum' (with a long 'mmm').
12 As hands come to rest in yoni mudra on belly, inhale and exhale 'ram' (with a long 'mmm').

Tips

The bija mantras can be practised as one long sound for length of exhalation, or lots of short sounds, as many as it takes to fill the length of exhale. For example, instead of sounding a single long 'yammm' with as many 'mmm's as is needed to reach end of exhale, instead voice a series of rapid sounds: 'yam, yam, yam, yam, yam' with as many short 'yams' as needed to reach end of breath. This practice also works well standing.

Punctuated golden thread exhalation with sankalpa (affirmations)

Sankalpa, meaning positive resolve, is a powerful element of mental practice in yoga. It is rather like an affirmation: a short statement in simple language that frames a positive goal or intention. Sankalpa is best expressed in the present tense, as if the future was now. This gives immediacy, and provides focus for an aim whose realization would bring great joy. Your sankalpa is a private matter, you choose it yourself, and it is often wisest to keep it secret. Traditionally, the sankalpa is repeated at the beginning and end of a deeply restorative meditation practice called yoga nidra (p. 166), but it can also be used, as described below, in the pauses of Punctuated golden thread breath.

Take time to frame a positive resolve that resonates with your intuitive higher wisdom. Reflect upon your priorities and your immediate and long-term aims before finally settling upon the right affirmation for you. Keep it simple and always use the same words and phrases whenever you repeat the sankalpa.

Traditionally, the sankalpa is made and repeated until it comes to fruition. A lofty, spiritually-elevating sankalpa might remain the same for a lifetime. But it is perfectly possible and quite practical to adopt sankalpas specifically appropriate to pregnancy, childbirth or post-natal recovery. These 'short-term' sankalpas serve to focus mental energy and can be encouraging and strengthening in the face of challenges or as a way to overcome fears and anxieties. Examples of sankalpas appropriate to pregnancy include: 'My every breath nourishes my baby', or 'I have everything I need to birth my baby'.

This practice works best when you feel that the silent inner voice speaking the sankalpa is voicing the wisdom you feel in your heart. Whilst it is helpful to have external encouragement from those around you, that silent inner voice is more powerful than any number of outer voices. The pauses along the breath in the following technique provide little islands of stillness in which you can repeat your sankalpa silently to yourself.

1 Follow instructions for Punctuated golden thread practice (p. 117).

2 Use whichever form of exhale–pause pattern you prefer: either straight thread, or corkscrew.

3 In each pause, hear a powerful silent inner voice from your own heart – a voice coming from a place of deep wisdom.

4 In all pauses along exhale, hear that inner voice repeating your sankalpa.

5 Choose something that resonates with your present need for encouragement, reassurance or compassion. For example, something simple like 'Be here now', 'Yes, be here now', a reminder to deal just with this present moment. Maybe the voice could remind you to take courage, and be strong in your knowledge that 'I can do it and the baby can'.

6 Hear the voice of your heart's wisdom repeating your sankalpa in pauses along the exhalation.

Tips

It can be helpful to perceive the first repetition of the sankalpa as planting a seed. Each time you repeat it, you nourish and nurture what you have planted.

If you are keen to imbue your sankalpa with spirited energy, you may want to use it in a number of different yoga practices in addition to hearing it repeated in pauses along the exhale. For example, it can mark your transition from one state of consciousness to another: by being the first thing in your mind upon awakening in the morning, and the last thing of which you have conscious awareness as you drift off to sleep. It can also be used at a specific point in each breath cycle when using a Full yogic breath (p. 13), or any rhythmic easeful breath practice, such as Ujjayi (p. 16), for example hearing it repeated on each exhalation, or placing it consciously at the transition between inhale and exhale.

A positive affirmation can be of great comfort and reassurance during any major challenge, such as childbirth. But whilst the sankalpa appears to be operating just at the level of having something to 'hang onto' during difficulty, in fact it works at a far deeper level than that. It is buried very deep into your subconscious mind, and works to transform your whole way of being and thinking by increasing your receptivity to intuitive wisdom and inner guidance. This potential for transformation is increased when the sankalpa is allied with the breath.

Yoga nidra

Audio CD track 5

Yoga nidra literally means 'yoga sleep', but paradoxically it fosters a more awakened state of consciousness in which wisdom naturally arises. It encourages the physical body to enter a deeply relaxed state, whilst freeing the mind from sensory input in order to access insights. In pregnancy, both deep rest and spontaneous access to wisdom and understanding are especially welcome benefits.

A full practice is included on audio CD track 5, and the best way to experience yoga nidra is simply to lie down and listen. However, it can be reassuring to know more about the technique before you do it, so the outline below describes the practice you can hear on the CD, and also gives instructions for getting the most benefit from it. Once you are familiar with yoga nidra, you can use this written outline to remind you of the key stages of practice so that you can do it for yourself, mentally, without listening to the CD.

Before you start to listen to the audio CD track, the most important preliminary for an experience of yoga nidra is total physical comfort. Choose a lying or restorative pose appropriate to your stage of pregnancy (pp. 34, 36 and 70) and have sufficient props and covers to be warm, well supported and absolutely comfortable. Dim lights, draw curtains or cover your eyes. If you are uncomfortable or chilly, or if it is bright, then the physical body will not relax so well or so deeply, and will provide distractions from the focus of the practice. To minimize distraction from the physical body, and to deepen the quality of rest experienced in yoga nidra you are usually advised to keep perfectly still throughout. However, in pregnancy this is not always a realistic option. So, for example, if the baby shifts or you have cramp, then do adjust your position, but with awareness.

Once the physical body is comfortable, begin to listen to the audio track. It starts with instructions to settle the physical body, and guidance on breath observation. As the body settles more completely, breath and heart rate will slow, although this process takes longer than usual in pregnancy.

As the slowing breath settles physical and energy bodies deeper into a resting state, you are invited mentally to repeat a practice-specific sankalpa to become receptive and attentive. If you prefer you can use your own sankalpa either instead of or in addition to this short-term resolve.

Mental attention is then guided around the physical body. At the end of this rotation of consciousness, you are asked to create contrasting imaginary physical experiences of heaviness and lightness, and then to direct the focus of mental attention to the mind's eye, where you are invited to see a visual image of your baby. The body of the baby is described as lying in optimal foetal position, and mental focus is guided around the baby's body, in the same way as awareness rotated around your own physical body.

After a time for silent communication between mother and baby, focus of attention is returned to the breath. The sankalpa is revisited and the sound of the breath is used as a link back to more everyday awareness. Physical reawakening is encouraged through gentle stretches, and the practice closes.

Tips

Spend as much time coming out of yoga nidra as you did settling into it. Do not rush to sit up. Savour the effects of the practice, and move slowly and gently out of your resting position. Give yourself enough time to readjust mentally as well as physically, and gradually make the transition of stillness to activity.

Inner silence (antar mouna)

The basis for this calming and nurturing breath and sensory awareness practice is a meditation from the tantras called Inner silence (antar mouna). Usually it is taught very formally, as a sequential progression of directed awareness leading to deeper enquiry and mental focus. For use during pregnancy, a more informal approach is appropriate, since it can easily be adapted to your changing needs. Even in this informal version the essential quality of the original inner silence meditation is accessed: a healing and restorative calm that promotes receptivity.

1 Sit or lie comfortably.
2 Slowly establish a Full yogic breath. If it feels right, close eyes, and if not, let them relax, cast down.
3 As breath comes in and out through nose, be aware of rhythmic cycle of breath. Allow this natural flow of breath to continue easily as you shift focus of mental attention from one sense to the next.
4 First bring full attention to the sense of hearing.
5 Exhale awareness into the sense of hearing and be aware of sounds around you. Notice sounds furthest away from you. Then notice sounds closest to you. Draw attention closer until you are just focusing upon the sound of your own

breath as it comes in and goes out. Listen to this intimate sound. Let each sound be recognized, and then pass on to the next. Give full attention to the sense of hearing.

6 Feel breath as it comes in and out.

7 Shift focus of mental attention to the sense of touch.

8 Exhale awareness into the sense of touch. Notice different temperatures and textures you can detect through the feeling skin. Be aware of different temperatures of covered skin, in comparison with uncovered skin. Be aware of temperature of breath as it travels across upper lip into nostrils, and as it leaves nostrils and flows across upper lip. Notice any movements of the baby inside. Let each touch sensation, its temperature, its texture, be recognized, and then pass on to the next. Give full attention to the sense of touch.

9 Be aware of breath travelling up into nostrils, and follow its path into body as far as your awareness permits. Then follow it out again. Next time breath comes back into nostrils, shift attention to the sense of smell. Be aware of all odours and aromas you can detect as breath comes in. Let each smell be recognized, and then pass to the next. Give full attention to the sense of smell.

10 Next shift awareness from nose to mouth, away from sense of smell to the closely-related sense of taste. Exhale awareness into the sense of taste. Become aware of different tastes experienced on surface of tongue. Notice which tastes seem most easily detectable right now, sweet, or sour, hot or salty, bitter or astringent, like vinegar? Let each taste be recognized, and then pass on to the next. Give full focus of attention to the sense of taste.

11 Then direct attention away from mouth, to eyes.

12 Exhale awareness into the sense of sight. With lids closed, or cast down, just rest with all interest at the relaxed eyes, and see what there is to be seen in front of them, colours or darkness, movement or stillness, patterns or random shapes? Whatever you see, just observe quietly and let the images pass. Give your full attention to the sense of sight.

13 Lastly, bring attention back to where you started, to the sense of hearing. Just notice the intimate sound closest to you: the sound of your own breath. Gradually begin to move attention outwards from this sound, to become aware of sounds in the room around you, sounds outside of that room, sounds of the wider world. Be aware simultaneously of sounds closest and sounds furthest away.

14 When you are fully aware of all the sounds, breathe a little deeper, take a yawn or two, and open eyes.

Tips

The mental attitude of dispassionate interest that this practice fosters is of such great value during pregnancy that it is worth developing in daily life. There is no need to set aside a special meditation time or place, you can use the essence of the practice to access your place of inner silence any time.

The Feeding breath (p. 219, **Audio CD track 6**) is a special version of this practice for the post-natal period that incorporates sensory awareness of the presence of the feeding baby. You can listen to the audio track of this practice during pregnancy, simply transposing the references to the 'feeding baby' to the baby growing inside you.

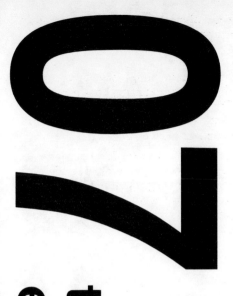

07

the joy body: ether/space

In this chapter you will learn:
- yoga practices to cultivate acceptance, praise, and gratitude that lead to joy
- how to combine practices to create your own yoga sequences
- yoga programmes to relieve common discomforts in pregnancy.

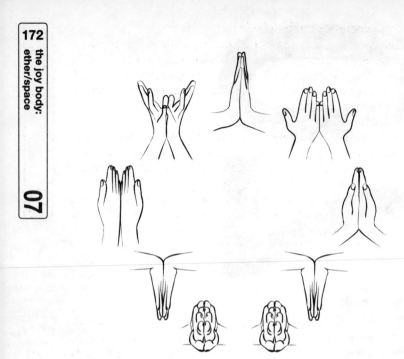

figure 7.1 Opening the mothering lotus

Opening the mothering lotus

This beautiful practice combines a fluid hand gesture sequence with bija mantras. It synchronizes sound, breath and movement to create a vivid experience of filling the heart with mother love. This promotes acceptance of abundance and joy.

The gestures are a manual metaphor of mothering experience. It begins with the lotus as a closed bud (palms together), moves through a period of upheaval, in which the bud is turned upside down, and inside out, to come to a pause where you have a moment to nurture yourself with an inhalation. After this moment of nurturing in the midst of upheaval, the closed bud returns to the heart space, transformed into a fully-blooming, open lotus. It is through the challenges and upheavals of mothering, which turn your life upside down and inside out, that your heart comes to open fully, and bloom with love for your child(ren).

1 Sit comfortably and breathe fully.

2 Inhale with hands in closed lotus position: palms together, fingertips pointing upwards, thumbs on breastbone.

3 Exhaling, move hands forward, rolling palms open as if opening the pages of a book (palms facing chest, with sides of little fingers touching).

4 Look down into the open palms/pages of the book.

5 Keep outsides of little fingers touching like the book's spine, and continue to open out palms, letting wrists turn and pivot against each other until backs of hands are touching and fingers point in towards you; elbows will move up and out to sides.

6 Keep pivoting wrists against each other with hands rotating inwards and down so fingertips point downwards. Now the start position has been turned upside down and 'inside out'.

7 Let hands keep turning, backs touching.

8 Keeping backs of hands together, turn wrists so fingertips point away; straighten elbows and stretch arms straight out at heart level, fingertips pointing forwards.

9 Pause and inhale deeply.

10 Exhaling, bend elbows and draw 'inside out' hands closer in, turning wrists so fingertips point straight down. Keep backs of wrists touching and continue exhaling as fingertips roll to point in towards body, turning wrists until fingertips point upwards.

11 Then open up the palms/pages of the book again.

12 Using meeting point between little finger sides as the spine of the book, roll palms back towards each other.

13 Bring hands into open lotus position: keeping two thumb sides touching, and maintaining contact between outer sides of two little fingers, stretch other fingers into as wide open a lotus bloom as you choose – anything from a barely open bud, with fingers close and bent, to an open bloom, with fingers straight, widely spaced and stretching away from each other.

14 This is one whole cycle of Opening the mothering lotus: inhale–exhale–inhale–exhale.

15 Practise until breath rhythm and movement pattern synchronize.

16 Then prepare to voice the breath.

17 Inhale with hands in closed lotus position: palms together, fingertips pointing upwards, thumbs resting on breastbone.

18 Exhaling, sound 'yam' as palms roll open, turning fingers down and out to bring hands 'inside out' with arms straight out in front.

19 Pause and inhale deeply.
20 Exhaling, sound 'yam' as elbows bend, drawing 'inside out' with hands closer in, turning wrists and forming open lotus at heart.

Tips

Opening the mothering lotus is a powerful practice because it embodies attitudes of receptivity and open-hearted embracing of change. If these attitudes are invited to live in your heart, then the gates to joy are wide open. To meet the demands of pregnancy, childbirth and mothering requires acceptance, compassion and great courage. Understanding the metaphor of this synchronized practice can invite these qualities into your life: the turning hands demonstrate the shifting upheavals (upside down and inside out) which it is necessary to accept; show that courage (whose root word is *cor* – Latin for heart) requires an open heart; and reveal that opening of the heart can be a blooming into maturity that allows for deep compassion and understanding.

Yoga perspectives on bliss

Bliss is the essential nature of the unity of consciousness, and this is the origin and aim of yoga practice. The intention of all yoga is to free the practitioner from suffering, to rest in a blissful state of pure being. In practical terms, yoga techniques can give you greater physical comfort through increased mobility and strength which leads to higher levels of vitality, a deeper sense of emotional stability and mental clarity that opens the doors to intuitive wisdom and provides clear guidance for wise choices in life. Ultimately though, all these impressive benefits are just side effects. But the side effects are so welcome that they tend to lead yoga practitioners towards at least a practical, human understanding of ananda (bliss): by accepting the benefits of your yoga practice, you develop an attitude of gratitude that leads naturally into experiences of deep appreciation and trust in the natural goodness and abundance of the universe. This understanding of the natural state of abundance and perfection is very clearly expressed in the following Sanskrit chant from the Upanisads, the 3,000 year-old Indian scriptures that provide the framework for this book.

Purnamadah purnamidam
Purnat purnamudacyate
Purnasya purnamadaya
Purnameva vasisyate

In translation, the chant says:

Everything in this, our inner world, is whole, complete
and perfect.
Everything in that, the outer world, is whole, complete
and perfect.
Everything that is whole, complete and perfect comes
from wholeness, completion and perfection itself,
and the original source of all this perfection simply
remains always perfect,
even though the entire, complete and perfect world
emerges from it.

In pregnancy, when the inner world is so clearly manifesting
abundance in the form of a new life, the sound and meaning of
this chant can have very deep resonance. Listening to or
chanting the words, and reflecting upon their meaning makes a
perfect conclusion to any yoga programme, and maximizes its
benefits.

Creating integrated yoga practice

**Putting it all together: fully integrated yoga practice for strength,
vitality, harmony and nourishment during pregnancy.**

The 'purnamada' chant uses sound, breath and meaning to
create an attitude of appreciative acceptance. The Opening the
mothering lotus sequence synchronizes breath, sound,
movement and meaning to promote understanding. Both are
integrated, synchronized practices, satisfying on many different
levels. The previous chapters provide basic ingredients for many
more such integrated practices of yoga in pregnancy, which can
be combined to create holistic programmes appropriate to your
needs. The primary breaths can be linked with individual asanas
from each base position described in Chapter 03; rhythmic
movements and breath awareness described in Chapter 04 can
be done in any base position to heighten awareness and free
movement in joints, releasing blocked energy, increasing vitality
and building strength. The sound work in Chapter 05 can be

incorporated with breath and mudras to add a further level of experience, and then these integrated practices can be followed with a period of stillness in any of the restorative poses in Chapter 03. Finally, the meditations and yoga nidra practices in Chapters 06 and 07 can be used either independently, or as the conclusion of a movement practice, to promote profound rest, healing and peace.

Even if you have limited time, it is always best to do a truly holistic practice that includes all of the following elements. Balanced proportions of each element are given below with suggested timings to help you plan your programme according to the time available, ranging from a short practice of 20 minutes, to a full 90-minute session, such as a teacher might provide in a class. If you are really pushed for time, and can only manage one element of the programme, then choose resting practices.

1 Centring and breath awareness, seated or lying (1–10 minutes).
2 Energizing rhythms/simple movement with breath (4–15 minutes).
3 Flowing sequence of movement with breath (4–15 minutes).
4 Synchronized practice with sound, breath, movement and gesture (2–10 minutes).
5 Restorative pose, possibly with yoga nidra or other meditation (8–30 minutes).
6 Closing practice to centre and focus (e.g. breath, sound, meditation) (1–10 minutes).

Perhaps the most challenging element of such a holistic programme is the creation of flowing and synchronized sequences. But once you are familiar with individual practices, then it is fairly easy to link together a coherent sequence if you observe a few wise cautions:

• Remember the ease of transition between poses.
• Respect your own limits.
• Know when to stop.
• Never allow your enthusiasm for the sequence you are following to compromise your attention to comfort.
• Always tune into the rhythm of breath, which should be easy and unforced.
• Be sure to stop *before* you reach the point of struggle or tiredness.

Within the safe boundaries marked by the observation of these cautions, there is creative joy to be had in making yoga sequences.

Flowing sequences of postures

There are several ways to link poses into useful sequences, and some examples are provided below.

Begin with the samples below, which connect poses from a range of different base positions, grouped together in a fluid flow. The three examples given are suitable for different levels of vitality and energy, so select the sequence that best matches your current needs. These are long sequences, so if you start to run out of energy, omit the optional poses marked *, or reduce the number of repetitions.

Sun salutation modification

For high vitality days.

This adapts a classic yoga sun salutation (surya namaskar) to provide more space, time and support for the pregnant body.

1	2	3	4
Mountain pose (p. 79) with Namaste and pelvic scoops (p. 81), three rounds of breath	Lift the spirits arms in standing three repetitions (p. 56)	Transition from standing to all fours (p. 28)	Cat inhale and exhale three repetitions (p. 39)
5	**6**	**7**	**8**
* Supported Cat lunge (left foot forward) (p. 45) with arm circles, three repetitions	Cat (p. 39)	*Half moon variation with right leg straight (p. 50) three rounds of breath	* Cat (p. 39)

9	10	11	12
* Half squat circles (left foot forward), three repetitions in both directions (p. 46)	Hare pose rest (as long as necessary) (p. 40)	Flowing Hare-to-cat swoop inhale and exhale, three repetitions (p. 42)	Transition from all fours to standing (p. 32)
13	**14**	**15**	**16**
Mountain pose (p. 79)	Lift the spirits arms (p. 56)	Mountain Pose (p. 55) Three rounds of breath in this pose.	Namaste (p. 55)

Pause, then repeat again with right foot forward in Cat lunge and Half squat circles, and right leg back in Half moon.

Moon sequence (Chandra namaskar)

For quieter, or medium vitality days.

Focused around the central point of the pelvis held steady in Cat lunge pose, this flow connects with gentle lunar energy. Because Cat lunge base is sustained for a while, put padding under knees.

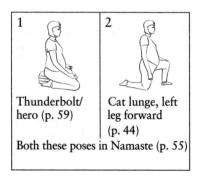

1	2
Thunderbolt/ hero (p. 59)	Cat lunge, left leg forward (p. 44)
Both these poses in Namaste (p. 55)	

3–6 All four poses below from Cat lunge family, left leg forward (p. 44)			
3 Cat lunge with Namaste quartet part one: open the heart (p. 55)	4 Cat lunge with Namaste quartet part two: lift the spirits (p. 56)	5 Cat lunge with Namaste quartet part three: reach with ease (p. 56)	6 Cat lunge Namaste quartet part four: build vitality (p. 57)
7 Cat inhale and exhale, three repetitions (p. 39)	8 *Cat-dog-cat parts one and two, up to to three repetitions (p. 51)	9 Hare pose rest (as long as necessary) (p. 40)	10 *Flowing hare-to-cat swoop inhale and exhale, three repetitions (p. 42)
11 Hare pose rest (as long as necessary) (p. 40)	12 Thunderbolt/ hero in Namaste (p. 59)		
Repeat whole sequence from Cat lunge, right leg forward.			

Standing flow

For days when you are feeling strong and vigorous.

This flow incorporates an opening and closing namaskaram (greeting) with squats, balances, and a range of warrior options to promote courage, strength and vitality.

1	2	3	4
Mountain pose with pelvic scoops and rocking (p. 79)	Squatting namaskaram (p. 92) Alternate between these two, three repetitions	Forward reach with earth blessing (p. 93)	Step right foot forward into Basic warrior stance (p. 105)

4	5	6	7
First warrior (p. 106) Alternate between these two arm positions, three repetitions, with optional pelvic circles	Second warrior (p. 107)	*Warrior of the heart, three rounds of breath (p. 109)	Step back into Squatting namaskaram (p. 92)

8	9	10	11
* Victory pose of the fierce goddess (p. 94) Alternate between these two, three repetitions	*Lord of the Dance (p. 95)	Squatting namaskaram (p. 92) Alternate between these two, three repetitions	Forward reach with earth blessing (p. 93)

For variation, substitute Fierce Goddess/Lord of the Dance alternation with:	Repeat whole sequence with left foot forward in Warriors, or for for a shorter sequence, change front position when alternating First and Second warriors.
Tree balance (p. 87)	and/or Heavenly stretch (p. 82)

When you feel comfortable with some of these sequences, and have experience with the individual practices in Chapters 02, 03 and 04, then let your creativity flow to devise your own posture sequences. Remember when linking postures to consider the ease with which you can move from one practice to the next, so incorporate the transitional moves (p. 27) when planning your sequences.

Depth from steadinesss

You can stick with a particular base pose in which you feel comfortable and play through the range of options accessible in that position. For example, any seated base provides an opportunity to explore most chest opening sequences, plus side and back bends, and twists and forward rest as described below.

Earthed seated flow

For quieter days when you feel heavier but require an energy boost.

Keeping steady and close to the ground, this flow nourishes depleted energy and encourages stability and security. For a shorter sequence, omit optional sequences marked * or reduce repetitions.

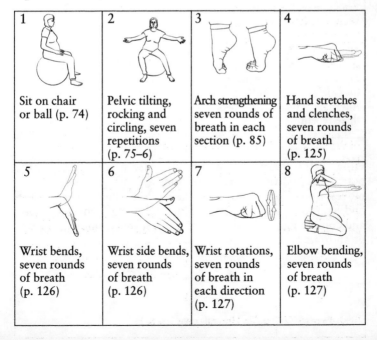

1	2	3	4
Sit on chair or ball (p. 74)	Pelvic tilting, rocking and circling, seven repetitions (p. 75–6)	Arch strengthening seven rounds of breath in each section (p. 85)	Hand stretches and clenches, seven rounds of breath (p. 125)
5	6	7	8
Wrist bends, seven rounds of breath (p. 126)	Wrist side bends, seven rounds of breath (p. 126)	Wrist rotations, seven rounds of breath in each direction (p. 127)	Elbow bending, seven rounds of breath (p. 127)

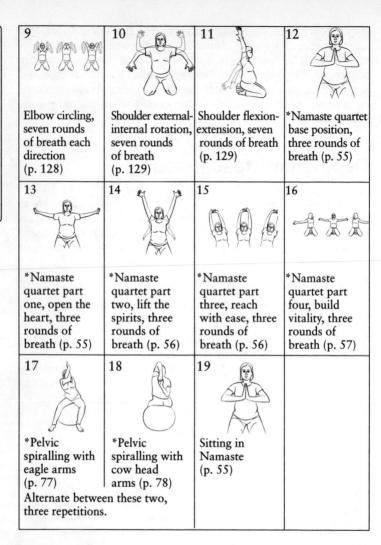

9	10	11	12
Elbow circling, seven rounds of breath each direction (p. 128)	Shoulder external-internal rotation, seven rounds of breath (p. 129)	Shoulder flexion-extension, seven rounds of breath (p. 129)	*Namaste quartet base position, three rounds of breath (p. 55)
13	**14**	**15**	**16**
*Namaste quartet part one, open the heart, three rounds of breath (p. 55)	*Namaste quartet part two, lift the spirits, three rounds of breath (p. 56)	*Namaste quartet part three, reach with ease, three rounds of breath (p. 56)	*Namaste quartet part four, build vitality, three rounds of breath (p. 57)
17	**18**	**19**	
*Pelvic spiralling with eagle arms (p. 77)	*Pelvic spiralling with cow head arms (p. 78)	Sitting in Namaste (p. 55)	
Alternate between these two, three repetitions.			

Other helpful combinations to consider when exploring the potential of particular base positions are: using all upper body moves with various seated positions, doing Energy freeing feet and leg moves and/or Energy block releasing from Stick pose, and combining pelvic movements with seated, standing, warrior or all fours bases.

Healing sequences for relief from pain or discomfort

If you have a particular health issue then you can follow the suggested yoga responses listed in the index, creating a mini sequence specifically to address your concern. Sample programmes for common experiences in pregnancy are provided below.

Lower back pain

To ease and prevent lower back pain.

This promotes fluid movement with the spine horizontal and vertical, and uses stabilizing poses to encourage balanced posture.

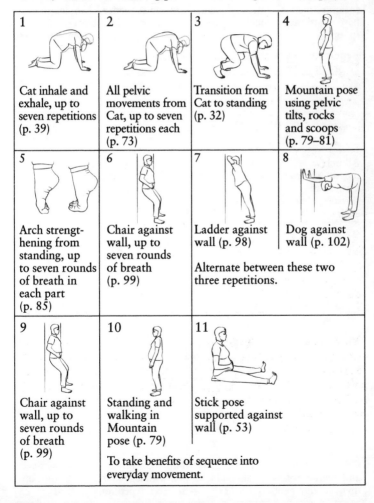

1	2	3	4
Cat inhale and exhale, up to seven repetitions (p. 39)	All pelvic movements from Cat, up to seven repetitions each (p. 73)	Transition from Cat to standing (p. 32)	Mountain pose using pelvic tilts, rocks and scoops (p. 79–81)
5	**6**	**7**	**8**
Arch strengthening from standing, up to seven rounds of breath in each part (p. 85)	Chair against wall, up to seven rounds of breath (p. 99)	Ladder against wall (p. 98) Alternate between these two three repetitions.	Dog against wall (p. 102)
9	**10**	**11**	
Chair against wall, up to seven rounds of breath (p. 99)	Standing and walking in Mountain pose (p. 79) To take benefits of sequence into everyday movement.	Stick pose supported against wall (p. 53)	

Pelvic pain

For prevention and management of pelvic pain and instability (pubis symphysis dysfunction and sacroiliac pain).

During all moves, use Golden thread exhalation (p. 18) and mula bandha (p. 139) to promote strong support from toning of pelvic floor muscles. Squeeze buttocks firmly together with every exhalation.

1	2	3	4
Sacral stabilization sequence base position (p. 63)	Sacral stabilization sequence, rocking (p. 65)	Sacral stabilization sequence, twisting (p. 66)	Cat inhalf and exhale, up to seven repetitions (p. 39)
Repeat this set of poses again on the other side before proceeding.			
5	6	7	8
All pelvic movements from Cat, up to seven repetitions each (p. 73)	Transition from Cat to standing (p. 32)	Mountain pose using pelvic tilts, rocks and scoops (p. 79–81)	Chair against wall, up to seven rounds of breath (p. 99)
9	10	11	12
Ladder against wall (p. 98)	Dog against wall (p. 102)	Chair against wall, up to seven rounds of breath (p. 99)	Stick pose supported against wall (p. 53)
Alternate between these two up to three times, up to seven rounds of breath in each			
13		14	
Only if no acute pain: Hip external and internal rotation right and left, up to seven repetitions (p. 123)		Hip adduction-abduction right and left with legs squeezed together, up to seven repetitions (p. 124)	

Heartburn and indigestion

For relief of heartburn and indigestion, and to free space in the upper back.

1	2	3	4
Side stretch against wall, alternate both sides three times, up to seven rounds of breath (p. 101)	Mountain pose (p. 79)	Transition to all fours (p. 28)	Thunderbolt/hero seat for as long as comfortable (p. 59), with Heart/womb breath (p. 145)
5	6	7	8
Namaste quartet part two, up to seven repetitions from Thunderbolt/hero seat or Stick Pose (p. 56)	Namaste quartet part three up to seven repetitions from Thunderbolt/hero seat or Stick Pose (p. 56)	Hare pose with high support (p. 40) Choose one of these options to close sequence	Restorative butterfly (p. 70)

Breathlessness

To relieve and prevent breathlessness.

1	2	3	4
Restorative butterfly (p. 70)	Air gesture (both hands) (p. 160)	Transition to all fours (p. 31)	Cat inhale and exhale (p. 39) with Ujjayi breath (p. 16)
Full yogic breath (Audio CD track 1) in this pose for as long as time permits.			

5	6	7	
Easy cross legged sitting (p. 62)	Spine extension-flexion up to seven rounds (p. 130) with Ujjayi breath (p. 16)	Stick pose (p. 53) or any comfortable seat with wall support if necessary for Prenatal sonic massage (p. 148–51)	

Swollen ankles and wrists

To ease tenderness of swollen and/or stiff wrists.

Proceed with gentleness and caution within comfort range if experiencing carpal tunnel syndrome. From any comfortable seated pose, Ujjayi breath with abdomiinal breath if possible (p. 16) for seven rounds of each of the following.

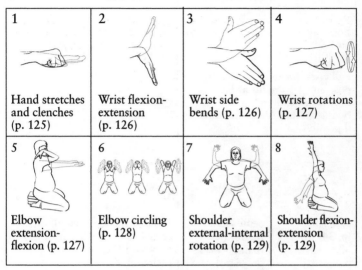

1	2	3	4
Hand stretches and clenches (p. 125)	Wrist flexion-extension (p. 126)	Wrist side bends (p. 126)	Wrist rotations (p. 127)
5	6	7	8
Elbow extension-flexion (p. 127)	Elbow circling (p. 128)	Shoulder external-internal rotation (p. 129)	Shoulder flexion-extension (p. 129)

To ease tenderness of swollen and/or stiff ankles.

Ujjayi breath with abdominal breath if possible (p. 16) for seven rounds of each of the following:

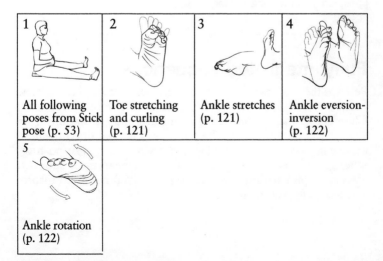

1	2	3	4
All following poses from Stick pose (p. 53)	Toe stretching and curling (p. 121)	Ankle stretches (p. 121)	Ankle eversion-inversion (p. 122)
5			
Ankle rotation (p. 122)			

Exhaustion

For exhaustion.

1	2	3	4
Restorative butterfly (p. 70)	Water gesture, both hands (p. 112)	Transition to all fours (p. 31)	Transition down to lying (p. 30)
Full yogic breath (p. 13) in this pose and gesture for as long as time permits, listening to yoga Nidra (p. 166, Audio CD track 5) if possible.			

5	6	
Side lying (p. 34) (over 30 weeks pregnant)	Semi-supine (p. 36) (less than 30 weeks pregnant)	Then, if vitality levels allow, complete Energy freeing series (p. 120–133), three rounds each with Full yogic breath (p. 13) or Ujjayi breath (p. 16)
Ujjayi breath in either of these poses (according to stage of pregnancy) for as long as time permits.		

Fully integrated sequences

Perhaps the most pleasing way to practise, once you have a basic familiarity with the instructions, is to integrate moves from Chapters 03 and 04 with sounds, attitudes and meditations from Chapters 05, 06 and 07. The hand gestures (mudras) from all these chapters can helpfully be incorporated into most postures where hands are not required for weight-bearing or support. Two examples with distinct effects are given below to inspire you to create your own integrations.

Heart-focused practice

For comfort and healing of mother and baby.

1	2	3	4
Warrior of the heart (p. 109) with rapid YAMMs on exhalation, three rounds in each leg position (left forward, then right forward)	Mountain pose (p. 79) Ujjayi breath (p. 16) in this pose for up to seven rounds.	Namaste (p. 55)	Transition to all fours (p. 28)

5	6	7	8
Half moon, right leg forward first, then left (p. 50) Right side first, then left side with cat inhale between two sides. Three rounds of breath each side	Heart gesture both hands (p. 142)	Cat inhale (p. 39)	Thunderbolt/ hero seat, three rounds of breath (p. 59)

9	10	11	
Namaste quartet part two lift spirits (p. 56) YAMM to resonate with energy of heart centre	Heart gesture both hands (p. 142)	Air gesture both hands (p. 161)	

Earth-focused practice

For stability and security.

1	2	3	4
Hare pose (p. 40) for Pelvic floor pranayama (p. 135–140) with Golden thread/Ujjayi breath (p. 118). Seven rounds of each.	Transition to sitting (p. 29)	Churning the mill (p. 134) with Golden thread breath (p. 16) seven rounds each direction	Stick pose (p. 53)
5	6	7	8
Namaste quartet part one (p. 55)	Namaste quartet part two (p. 56)	Namaste quartet part three (p. 56)	Namaste quartet part four (p. 57)

For all four above, both hands in Earth gesture (p. 21). Ujjayi breath (p. 16) and LAMM on every exhale to connect with energy of earth centre.

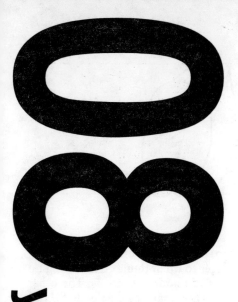

08

yoga for birth

In this chapter you will learn:
- how yoga can help you and your baby prepare for birth
- yoga practices to promote a relaxed attitude of acceptance during labour
- yoga movement and breath to birth more comfortably.

Apana mudra

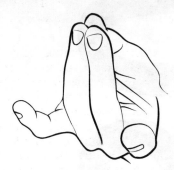

figure 8.1 Apana mudra

With hands resting palms up, comfortably on knees or thighs, lightly touch tip of middle finger to tip of thumb. Then bring tip of ring finger to join thumb and middle fingertips. The other fingers are relaxed. Hands are traditionally held palm up for this mudra, but if it feels easier, turn them over. This hand gesture connects to the downward moving flow of energy in the body, the current that controls functions such as urination, defecation and the flow of menses and semen. It is also the energy that powers the contractions of the uterus during labour and the birth of the baby. The mudra can be used to develop a sense of how this energy operates in your body, using core breaths described in Chapter 02, or during postures and movements in Chapters 03 and 04. If you find it comfortable, it can be helpfully applied during first stage labour, whilst using breathing practices or birthing positions described later in this chapter. It is also a useful gesture when you feel blocked, or unable to release, either physically (for example, if you are constipated) or emotionally (for example, if you feel choked up or suffocated by certain feelings or circumstances).

Yoga perspectives on childbirth

In the first chapter, you learnt that yoga meant 'union'. All the practices of yoga lead from and back to the unity of all things, and this understanding can promote a profoundly trusting open-heartedness. The intention of each practice described in all previous chapters is to encourage the mind to rest in the present moment, responding to every current experience as an expression of unity, without reference to the past or expectations about the future. By far the most powerful help that yoga has to offer you and your baby in labour is this attitude of openness and acceptance.

Giving birth can be an experience which women often describe as being 'out of time'; and so this yogic way of being fully in the present is particularly appropriate to meet the demands of childbirth. No one can plan what sort of labour she will have, and even less how she will respond to it. It is wise not to believe people who claim this kind of planning is possible, but it is prudent to invest time and effort in preparation for the unpredictable. The physical postures and moves which you have learnt may certainly enable you to labour more comfortably, and yoga's breath and sound practices can provide a powerfully effective approach to the management of pain and panic, but without doubt it is the internal awareness of unity, the open state of mind and heart which yoga fosters that will be of the most profound practical assistance at this time. At an intellectual level, it can also be reassuring to inform yourself about what you may expect during labour by attending antenatal classes in pregnancy (p. 235).

There are two key yoga techniques that are particularly helpful to practise in pregnancy to promote a positive, open frame of mind and calm focus during labour: the first is sankalpa or positive affirmation (p. 165), and the second is trataka, a combination of breath and focus (p. 153). Whilst appropriate yoga breath and movement can vary between different stages of labour, these two practices are invaluable throughout the whole process. To get maximum benefit it is best to practise them as often as you can during pregnancy.

Although traditionally sankalpa is a resolve that may be kept for years, or even a whole lifetime, it can be useful to devise a short-term affirmation specifically for use during pregnancy and labour. Examples of positive resolves that are helpful during labour include: 'Rest in every breath'; 'I know that I have everything I need to birth my baby'; 'Be here now' or 'Every contraction is one closer to meeting my baby'. Choose an affirmation that resonates deep in your heart, and it can carry you through labour.

The standard practice of trataka can be helpfully adapted for use during labour by combining focused gaze with directed breath to maintain a state of restful focused awareness, especially helpful as contractions increase in intensity. There is some debate about the importance of the image upon which you focus during this practice: some people are fussy, and others say it does not matter what you gaze at. The wisest approach is to use whatever is convenient and easily seen. If eyes are open during first stage labour, then it can be particularly reassuring to fix the gaze on the eyes of the birthing companion, and feel the breath bringing you into the support they offer. This becomes particularly powerful if you breathe together (Entrainment breathing, p. 157).

The combination of outer (eyes open) and inner (eyes closed) trataka with Golden thread breath (p. 18) works well if synchronized with the rhythm of contractions to create a natural pattern of outwards and inward gazing. Such a pattern can lead your focus inside during deep rest periods between contractions, and take your focus out to those around you at the peak of the contraction itself, or vice versa. What is important is to explore how you respond to the practice during pregnancy, and then adopt whichever version feels right during labour.

Stages of labour

Every woman's labour is different, and each birth has its own distinctive characteristics and quality. Birthing experiences may diverge dramatically from expectations and plans formed during pregnancy, and will very likely differ from previous births experienced by the same woman. However, across the broad spectrum of birth experiences, it is common to recognize three or four stages of labour, each with their own rhythm of contractions. The outline below describes briefly the common patterns in normal physiological labour.

In the first stage, particularly for women who have not previously experienced labour, a 'latent' stage often precedes a period of fully-established labour. During this 'latent' time, and indeed through the end of late pregnancy, the cervix is preparing to open: its softening is often described as 'ripening' and any contractions are likely to be erratic, stopping and starting with no particular pattern, sometimes for a short period, but sometimes over a few days or nights. For many women on their first labour this can be the longest stage. In established first stage labour, regular rhythmic contractions of the uterine muscles cause the cervix to further thin and open or dilate. It is during the second stage, once the cervix is fully dilated, that strong contractions help the baby to move down and out of the womb, through the birth canal and into the world. Many midwives also recognize the transition between first and second stage labour as a stage in itself, and others feel that any pause after full dilation and before the big second stage contractions which birth the baby is also a distinct phase of labour, and refer to this time as the 'rest and be thankful' stage. The third (or fourth) stage of labour is when the placenta is born. The relative proportions of time which may be spent in any given stage is entirely individual, and unpredictable, but in general, first stage is often at least four times longer (sometimes a much as ten times longer) than second stage, which can last anything from a few minutes to a few hours. The action of birthing the placenta is brief, and frequently hastened by management through certain drugs, but in a physiological (unmanaged) third stage there may be a pause of up to an hour before the placenta emerges.

A more comfortable labour with yoga

The baby during birth

One of the key factors determining the length and comfort of each stage of labour, and the number of contractions needed to birth your baby, is the position of the child in the womb. The term 'optimal foetal positioning' describes a baby who is best placed to take the easiest and quickest route into the world. Whilst it is generally agreed that the best position is for the baby to be head down, spine resting outwards into the curve of their mother's belly, there is some debate about the possibilities of encouraging babies into such positions during late pregnancy (for further reading on this topic see p. 231). It is encouraging to know, however, that amongst those people who believe that maternal posture in late pregnancy and labour *can* help babies to adopt and maintain 'optimal foetal position', many of the recommended poses and movements for mothers are very common in yoga practice. For example, spending time in Cat (p. 39), and Hare pose (p. 40), or pelvic rocking (p. 75) may all contribute to the likelihood of a well-positioned baby and a more comfortable labour. These positions are described below as appropriate yoga moves for use in labour and as birthing positions.

Yoga movements for labour and birth

The main value of yoga based movements during labour and birth is that they empower you to move with ease and confidence, because you have learnt to respect your body's natural range of motion and to be aware of your own comfort levels. These benefits come most readily if regular practice of yoga has built strength and encouraged mobility throughout pregnancy. The movements described below are not new inventions specifically for labour, but familiar poses that may have been used throughout pregnancy. Even if you are coming to them fairly late in pregnancy, just a little practice can be of benefit during labour.

Every labour is different, and often different stages of labour require distinct movement strategies to promote comfort and ease. The poses listed below are suggestions only, and not a prescriptive schedule. What matters most is that you move freely and appropriately during the different stages of your labour. Given this freedom to move and the embodied familiarity of the yoga poses, your body will instinctively adopt the best positions for you.

Yoga breath patterns for labour and birth

There is some debate about the value of breathing techniques during childbirth. Many midwives and childbirth educators argue that the only useful breath during labour is the pattern which the woman in labour adopts instinctively, and that learnt techniques are merely confusing distractions. Ideally, indeed, instinctive birthing breath does not need to be taught; in practice, however, instinctive behaviour of any kind is very alien to many women. Our lives have often become so far removed from what is natural and instinctive that many people's breathing patterns (shallow, choppy and erratic) are inimical to health and well-being. If this is true in daily life, it is clear that during an experience as intensely powerful as that of giving birth, some prior guidance may be needed to enable reconnection with instinctive and positive breathing patterns. This is why pranayama learnt and practised in pregnancy can be helpful during childbirth.

For yoga breathing to be of any real practical use during childbirth, it needs to have been practised sufficiently regularly during pregnancy to have become second nature, a living part of your embodied knowledge. In this way methods of yoga breathing cease to be simply 'learnt techniques' needing to be consciously recalled, but are so deeply embedded in the unconscious that they actually promote an instinctive approach to breath in labour. In fact, as you may have discovered, many of the core yoga breaths are not 'techniques' as such, but are in fact based upon the natural physiology of complete breathing patterns, so are often more deeply instinctive to the body than the habitual patterns of incomplete or shallow breath that have been adopted in response to stress or tension.

The complete and relaxed breathing patterns encouraged by the practice of yoga are of particular benefit to manage the pain of contractions, but it is also worth knowing that these same breaths provide pain management for other experiences, for example post-caesarean recovery, during after-pains, or during healing following episiotomies or tears.

During labour, breath works most effectively as a system of pain management when you rest completely between contractions. Your body will move in whatever way is comfortable during contractions, but between them you need to be sure to rest easily. Return to Ujjayi (p. 18), or Golden thread exhalation (p. 16), or whatever breathing pattern helps you to relax completely in the spaces between contractions. Remember it is the rest *between* that is the key to being prepared to cope well when the next contraction comes.

There are absolutely no rules about breathing for pain management in labour and there is certainly no single correct approach to the application of pranayama during childbirth. In physiological terms, it is the exhalation which is the antidote to pain: slow, complete exhales reduce heart rate, encourage full inhalation to maintain optimum oxygen levels for mother and baby, and induce a state of calm. So it makes sense to focus on exhalation during labour, in whatever way feels natural to you. If you can do this, then some version of Golden thread exhalation will probably arise quite spontaneously.

The following section offers a range of practices which many women have found helpful in labour. Each individual will discover her own particular rhythm of breath, and make use of the practices in the way most appropriate to her own birthing experience. That said, as a general guide, it is helpful to consider yoga breathing for childbirth both in relation to the labour stages at which it is likely to be relevant, and in relation to the physical movements which may be most helpful at each stage. This is the order in which they appear below.

Cautions

If you are planning to make use of any yoga breaths in labour, it is worth informing (or asking your birth companion to inform) the attending midwives about what you are doing. Let them know that sometimes these practices work so effectively that the resultant ability to cope with pain may give a misleading impression about the intensity of the contractions that you are experiencing or the stage of dilation you have reached.

In each section below, the list of practices is followed by tips to help you tailor techniques already described elsewhere in the book for use in labour and birth. Practices appearing for the first time are described in full.

Pre-labour (latent stage)

Useful yoga breaths:

- Circle of breath (p. 11)
- Full yogic breath (p. 13, **Audio CD track 1**)
- Golden thread exhalations and variants (p. 16, **Audio CD track 3**)
- Entrainment breath (p. 157)
- Ujjayi (if it can be done effortlessly) (p. 18, **Audio CD track 2**).

Useful yoga poses and movements:

- Lateral lying with support (p. 34)
- Restorative butterfly (p. 70)/Hare pose rest with support (p. 40)
- Rhythmic pelvic rocking in Cat (p. 39)
- Ladder against wall (p. 98).

Tips

The main thing at this stage is to conserve energy and build resources in case labour turns out to be long. The physical postures should be well supported to provide comfortable rest for the physical body, and this rest is deepened by conscious use of breath. Whether you prefer to rest forwards (Hare pose) or backwards (Restorative butterfly) will probably depend upon the position of your baby. If you choose lateral lying, then be on your left side.

Full yogic breath in labour
Audio CD track 1

At the onset of labour, 'breathe for two'. Let a comfortable flowing Full yogic breath be your priority and it will calm and energize, building strength for labour. It can be helpful and reassuring to involve a birth partner with the rhythm of this breath by having them direct the focus into the upper back, where most breath movement happens during late pregnancy. To do this, be sitting or lying, and have your birthing partner sit down behind you, close enough to rest their hands on your upper back as you practice full yogic breath. Have the partner's hands completely relaxed and flat, with palms towards bottom of shoulder blades and fingertips pointing up. It should feel as if you are breathing into the warmth of the hands on your back. Let your birth companion breathe along with you, following the pace of your breath (Entrainment breath p. 157). The physical contact and shared breathing patterns promote a comforting form of non-verbal communication between you and your birthing companion. You feel the warmth of the supporting hands on your back and you also know that your partner is breathing with you.

Ujayii during labour

Audio CD track 2

This is a powerful tool to use at times during labour when you need to gather your resources and settle into yourself more. If you find Ujjayi comfortable and effortless, then it can be used throughout labour to bring you into a state of profound relaxation. However, you can just use it between contractions, when its soporific effects are especially helpful to promote deep rest. In this way, it is possible to alternate Ujjayi with Golden thread breath; using Ujjayi in rest periods, and Golden thread during contractions. It is also possible to combine Ujjayi with other breaths, as described in the next section.

Golden thread exhalation in labour

Audio CD track 3

During first stage labour, this is the breath that can ease most effectively through the contractions. Many women find it helpful to visualize the golden thread of breath as pulling them safely through the contractions, which can be seen either as steep mountains, where the breath helps you over each peak, or as ocean waves, with the golden thread guiding you over the crest of each wave.

Established first stage labour

Useful yoga breaths:

- Golden thread exhalations and variants (p. 16, **Audio CD track 3**)
- Peaks and valleys/Ocean waves breath (p. 202, **Audio CD track 4**)
- Entrainment breath (p. 157)
- Breath and focus (p. 153)
- Ujjayi (if it can be done effortlessly) (p. 18, **Audio CD track 2**).

Useful yoga poses and movements:

- Lateral lying with support (p. 34)
- Hare pose rest with support (p. 40)
- Hare pose rest with sacral massage (see figure below where partner rests palms on flat of lower back, providing still pressure or soothing strokes)

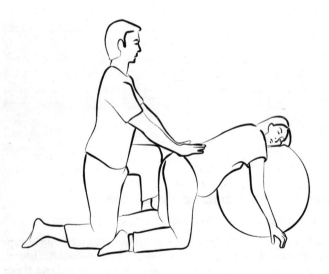

figure 8.2 Hare pose rest with sacral massage

- Restorative kneeling over ball (p. 61)
- Rhythmic pelvic rocking in Cat (p. 39)
- Seated forward rest (p. 71)/Double chair sitting (p. 72)
- Ladder against wall with pelvic movements (p. 98)
- Ladder against wall facing partner in Chair against wall (pp. 98 and 99), rest facing partner with your hands around their neck
- Supported squat (p. 91) (keep pelvis higher than knees at this stage, to encourage open pelvic inlet)
- Walking pelvic scoops (p. 81)
- Camel walking. (This is an adaptation of walking pelvic scoops, in which the scooping movement of the lower back is rolled up through the length of the spine, to the neck. Roll knees outwards as they lift, opening space in pelvis.)

Tips

The movements listed above include both supported resting and more active, upright postures. The most instinctive movement pattern during labour is often a progressive descent towards the floor: the upright, walking and shallow squatting options may be helpful during earlier first stage labour, when energy is high, but resting, quieter options may become more appropriate as labour progresses. If you find it more helpful to be upright, then Ladder against wall (p. 98), either alone or with a partner, can be a helpful place to rest between contractions. The upright, squatting and walking options are helpful if labour is slow to establish, or contractions seem to be lessening. The forward resting options are helpful for resting between contractions, or to help manage pain if contractions feel especially strong. Having a birth partner massage or simply bring firm still pressure to the sacrum during or between contractions while you rest forward can be very comforting.

Punctuated golden thread exhalation

This can be especially helpful during this stage of labour. It keeps the mind focused outside the body, and the extended out-breath gives the physical body a chance to come into its resting and relaxed mode between contractions. Conscious but easeful continuation of exhalation also promotes acceptance of each contraction. Since Golden thread works well in any position, including lying down in bed, if you find yourself labouring well in a side-lying resting position there is no need to move, just use this breath in whatever resting position you find most comfortable. If you find that at this stage in your labour you are more comfortable upright and walking about, then use the breath as you move.

You may discover, if you use this breath for a long time, that the size of the golden thread changes. For example, it may begin as a very fine thread, but grow thicker, transforming itself from thread to string, to skipping rope, until it resembles the heavy steel hawsers that moor gigantic ferryboats to port walls. Let such transformations occur naturally, for the basic method is just a starting point, and once you are familiar with it, then you can create whatever you need from what you have learnt.

Peaks and valleys/Ocean waves breath

Audio CD track 4

This provides a visual metaphor for a 'breathing journey'. It helps you shift between periods of rest and pain management, and is specifically helpful during first stage contractions. The description of the breathing journey gives you a feel for the patterns of contractions and pacing of breath characteristic of this stage of labour. The instructions are not intended as a set script, rather they show how breath can encourage an instinctive response to cope with pain.

The full instructions on the CD lead you through a series of imaginary contractions, whose mountainous summits and valleys, or towering peaks and troughs of ocean waves are matched by changing patterns of breath. Below is a brief outline of the audio track, to enable you to practise without listening to the CD.

1 Begin with slow, even, Golden thread exhalations (p. 18). Close eyes.

2 Imagine you are about to experience a contraction, a big surge of uterine energy. Use Golden thread exhalations to release any tension associated with your response.

3 Sense that the intensity of the contraction builds to a mountain peak or wave crest, with most powerful sensations at the top, and the quietest place of rest (at start and end of contraction) in the valley, or in the still quiet trough between waves.

4 At the start, in the valley, or in the still waters between the waves, exhalations can be long and smooth.

5 Let the thread of exhaling breath lead you up the slopes and over peak, or up from the trough and towards crest of next wave.

6 Each time you get to the end of the exhalation, settle back into your resting place, down in the valley, or in the still waters between the waves, where you are ready to take your next breath.

7 As contractions build in intensity, it may become more difficult to exhale for long. Even so, each time allow exhalation to lead you up the steeper slopes as intensity increases.

8 It will be harder now to exhale back down to the resting place.

9 Use the exhale like a rope, to pull you up and over the peaks or the tops of the waves, to guide you through the intensity. Know that every contraction is one closer to meeting your baby.

10 Once over the top, start moving down the other side – sensations will still be intense, and breaths may still be short, almost like panting at this stage, but focus on lengthening the exhale.

11 Know that the Golden thread breath is leading you down the mountain, or down into the trough between the waves.

12 Let exhalations grow longer as you return to the state of rest that begins and ends each contraction, sinking back down to the peaceful valley, or to the quiet space between the waves, the place where you find all your resources.

13 Down in that place of rest, let go of the Golden thread breath and return to effortless Ujjayi (p. 16), its sound marking the end of this stage of the journey.

14 Keep Ujjayi, if it feels comfortable, for the whole period of rest between contractions. When next contraction is imminent, shift back to Golden thread breath to lead you up over the mountains or the waves to continue your journey to the next rest space.

Transition

As for first stage: use yoga breaths, poses and movements according to comfort and inclination.

Second stage labour: birthing the baby

Useful yoga breaths:

- Ujjayi (as above) (p. 16, **Audio CD track 2**)
- Voiced exhalations (p. 206).
- Birthing breath as described below.

Useful yoga poses and movements for birth positions:

- Cat (p. 40)
- Cat lunge (p. 44)
- Half squat circle base (p. 46)
- *Supported half squat circle base (see figure below where partner kneels or sits facing you to provide support for your upper body)

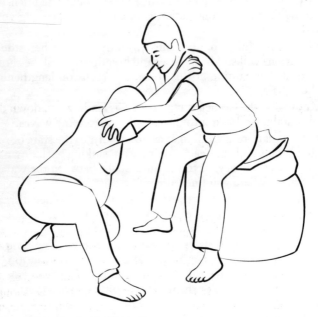

figure 8.3 Supported half squat

- Restorative kneeling (p. 61)
- Supported squat (p. 91)
- Supported squat with partner behind (see figure overleaf where partner sits behind you to provide support for your upper body)

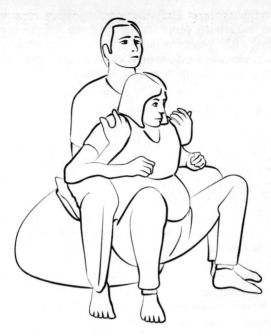

figure 8.4 Supported behind squat

- *Lateral lying with leg support (p. 34) (partner takes weight of upper leg on shoulder)
- Seated forward rest (p. 71)/Double chair sitting (p. 72).

Tips

The postures described above enable you to find the most comfortable position in which you can maintain an open pelvis for ease of birthing. All of these positions can be used throughout second stage labour right through to birth, except for the two sitting postures, from which you would need to rise once your baby is on the way out. If your second stage is longer than 20 minutes or so, you may prefer to move through a range of different birthing positions, both for your own comfort, and to provide shifts and changes to position that may encourage the baby to make the final part of their journey more easily.

All the postures are just the same as those described for practise during pregnancy, except for those marked *, which need additional support from a birthing partner. In these cases, it is well worth experimenting during pregnancy with your birthing partner to find the most comfortable arrangements for your body types, size and relative proportions. In all options, pelvic rocking and circling make positions more open and comfortable, whilst the breaths described below help you to work effectively with second stage contractions to birth your baby.

Voiced exhalations

In terms of birth preparation, finding a comfortable way to voice pain can be a vital tool in the relief of tension and panic. It is as if the sound on the breath carries pain away, and frees you to cope with the next contraction. Such sounding often occurs spontaneously during second stage labour, and can be a powerful tool for directing effort and focus. Whereas tight throated anxious screaming does little to relieve pain (it often increases the fear that intensifies experiences of pain), open throated sounds can release tension and manage pain. Practice the natural soundings to release (p. 147), whilst trying out the birthing positions, and you are more likely to be open to whatever sounds may come at this time. In particular, the Birthing breath can be more effective if throat and lips are soft and exhalation is voiced, so it is good to practice the instructions below with whatever sound feels natural.

Birthing breath

This breath is for use during second stage labour, to 'breathe the baby down' through the birth passage. It empowers you as a birthing mother to connect your breath with the movement of the baby, and to use your breathing patterns to maximize the effects of the second stage contractions. The Birthing breath combines pelvic floor awareness (p. 135) with focused directional breathing. To have a full understanding of the effect of this breath you need to be familiar with the pelvic floor practices first. Once you have learnt this breath then it is best to practise in the birthing positions you find most comfortable, but to begin, just sit comfortably and close eyes.

1 Use Golden thread exhalation (p. 18). If you feel comfortable with sound, let sounds come.

2 Keep breath flowing easily, moving attention up body on inhalation and down body on exhalation.

3 Rhythmically lift and lower pelvic floor: with each inhale, lift, and with each exhale, lower, connecting a sense of complete release with exhale.

4 Direct most of the downward exhalation to move awareness through the vagina, as if you were actually breathing out through it, tracing path of the baby's exit route.

5 Focus more attention upon exhale and release: the inhale is merely to enable you to exhale and release.

6 The exhale is always working with the contraction to breathe the baby out. You are literally breathing the baby down.

7 Second stage contractions could be around a minute long. You cannot exhale for a whole minute, so instead use a series of exhalations and pauses to work with contractions.

8 Some women find it helpful to imagine a cafetiere, a coffee pot with a plunger, its litre capacity marked up in 100 millilitre sections like a measuring jug, so you can pace your breath through the length of the contraction. Your body is the coffee pot, the baby is the coffee, and your breath is the plunger, exhaling down towards pelvic floor. But there is no bottom on the jug, so the baby comes right out at the end.

9 Breathe in, then exhale and release downward pressure, just a little bit down towards the pelvic floor. If you are using coffee pot plunger image, it will have descended only about one-tenth of the way down.

10 Then allow downward pressure of breath to remain at lowest point to which your awareness has reached, before breathing back in, and then continuing downward pressure with next exhalation from where you left off.

11 Keeping pressure there, inhale.

12 Each exhalation takes plunger further down coffee pot to the bottom, maintaining downward pressure as you breathe the baby out.

13 Inhale, and with next exhale, carry breath lower as you bear down, lengthening exhalation to feel further release in pelvic floor.

14 As pelvic floor releases at the end of last exhalation, direct your breath down and out through the vagina, following the path that the baby will take.

Tips

For practice during pregnancy, it can be helpful to feel that the muscles of the pelvic floor lift and squeeze on the inhalation, and then lower and release during exhalation. In this way, you can learn to associate the exhaling breath with the sense of release and softness that creates the opening necessary for the smooth journey of the baby through the birth passage.

The word most commonly used to describe second stage labour is 'pushing', with the implication that it involves force, effort and, crucially, a holding or 'blocking' of the breath. Whilst holding the breath *in* is not helpful, holding the breath *out* and pushing down towards the pelvic floor can indeed be a very helpful if the baby seems not to be coming down very fast, or where there are concerns about the baby's health, and a need to hurry the baby out. However, not all second stages need this approach all the time. In fact, the language of 'pushing' can sometimes more helpfully be translated into 'breathing the baby out', which is exactly what the Birthing breath does. There is no holding of the breath (in or out), just exhaling through a relaxed mouth. The downward and outward pressure which births the baby in this kind of breath all comes from reflex contraction of uterine muscles, without engaging more effortful downward pressure when the exhalation is blocked. Sometimes both kinds of breath are useful: more effortful 'pushing', and softer 'breathing the baby down'. It is important to know the difference and to be able to make the appropriate choice at the right time. Learning yoga practices like the pelvic floor techniques (p. 135) and the Birthing breath during pregnancy gives you an embodied understanding of your options in second stage labour.

Third stage labour: birthing the placenta

Useful yoga breaths:

- Full yogic breath (p. 13, **Audio CD track 1**)
- Birthing breath (as above)
- Golden thread exhalations and variants (p. 18, **Audio CD track 3**).

Useful yoga poses and movements:

- Restorative butterfly (p. 70).
- Supported squat with partner behind (p. 205) (partner sits behind you to provide support for your back).

Tips

The two suggested postures both provide supported rest after the effort of birthing, and enable you to feed your baby. The baby's suckling encourages a more rapid arrival of the placenta.

At this time, Restorative butterfly does not require usual amount of propping. Birthing breath (p. 206) can also be used to birth the placenta, but often a simple Ujjayi or Golden thread exhalation is sufficient.

Testimonies

These four inspiring accounts are from women who learnt the yoga described in this book during their pregnancies. Each birth was different, and each woman adapted what she had learnt to suit her own needs. There are page references for each of the practices they used.

Case study – Anna

Anna, who had practiced yoga for some years before she started pregnancy yoga classes, wrote about the birth of her son: 'I birthed Max, my second child, in the corridor of the birth centre at the Royal Women's Hospital in Brisbane, Australia, after a relatively short and joyful labour. We had just stepped into the building and I felt his head emerging. He weighed 9 lbs 1 oz (4.1 kg) and the labour was a joy. I went into labour gently in the early hours of the day Max was born, aware of strong but gentle contractions in my sleep. The most important thing I did was breathe and relax for as long as I could. I breathed deep into my belly to meet the contraction and let the sensation go on the out-breath (pp. 13 and 18). When the contractions became more intense at around 8 a.m. I began to move gently with them, the Cat pose (p. 40) provided great comfort and rest. I used this pose in the early stages of both of my labours quite extensively – just hanging out on the bed on all fours rising in and out with the contractions. My own take on Camel walking (p. 201) was also immensely helpful throughout the labour.

For this second labour the most important practice for me (along with the breath) was meditation (p. 163). Second time around I had complete trust in my body to be able to open and allow the baby through. My mind needed to trust and step out of the way (p. 19). I had read just prior to going into labour the physical effect of fear on the contractions and I meditated on trusting in the great wisdom of nature and of my body as part of nature. I had written in big letters the words "relax, let go, trust, breathe" and stuck it to the wardrobe in my bedroom. They became my mantra (sankalpa, p. 165) through the labour and brought huge resonance and relief.

I also got deeply into my intuitive self by focusing on my 'third eye' and moving from there (trataka, p. 153). When I felt the intense sensation of the cervix pulling up to allow the baby's head through I began to talk to my baby, half-singing, beseeching, wooing the little being through my body (p. 149). When he swam – or almost dived out! – I was standing, I put my hands down to feel his head emerging and scooped up his hot, wet, slippery body as he arrived. I felt ecstatic and empowered and now I try to remember to "relax, let go, trust and breathe" at all times!'

Case study – Frankie

Frankie is a yoga teacher with many years experience. She writes about the labour that led to the caesarean birth of her first daughter: 'I had a very long pre-labour (three days) with Lola. During this time I found it impossible to sleep. Yoga poses helped me to cope. I remember doing a lot of leaning forward over sofas/against walls during contractions (p. 72), and circling my hips (p. 75). I also spent a lot of time in a birthing pool, resting against the side in wide-kneeling stances (p. 61), and during contractions moving into half squats (p. 46). I focused on breathing out and keeping my jaw/throat soft, allowing sounds to come (p. 147).

Eventually however, as I got more and more tired, I realized I was starting to resist the contractions and it was much harder to focus on a soft breath. In a way, perhaps the most profound lesson of yoga during my experience of Lola's birth was how hard I found it to go with the flow when the flow didn't meet my expectations. It was humbling to have such a different experience from the one and I had hoped and planned for, and yet it was also amazing that my body was keeping going so long without sleep and for protecting her throughout all the intervention I ended up having. I realized I had reserves of strength and energy I hadn't known about and also the capacity to heal from the experience.'

Case study – Jessamie

Jessamie came to yoga for the very first time in the mid-stage of her first pregnancy: 'The yoga classes helped me to shed the anxiety I had about the birth itself, and shift my attention to an inner wisdom and innate understanding of what I was experiencing (p. 162). This transformation felt very profound and enabled me to feel more at one with myself and the baby, and more confident about having an enjoyable and uncomplicated pregnancy and birth. On a practical level, I switched from focusing solely on a hospital birth to aiming for a home birth instead. This was primarily because I let go of the fear I'd had regarding the pain of childbirth and the baby's safety, and embraced the positives of being at home in a more natural environment. I felt confident that we would be fine, and that this was a very special time.

During Charlie's birth, the breathing (p. 196) was an immensely powerful tool. It helped me to deal confidently with the contractions and allowed me to take myself off into my own space. It was reassuring too in that these methods had been shared with me because they had helped lots of other women in the past, and that gave me the confidence to embrace the whole experience in a very positive spirit and really connect with the sense that this was a very natural and wonderful time. I used my breath so that the contraction was like a wave (p. 202); I could sense it building up and this was my cue to find a comfortable position, for my partner Simon to rub my lower back, and for me to really focus on long exhalations, my version of the Golden thread (p. 18). The image I had in my mind was that I was blowing into the sails of a tiny ship as it crossed stormy waves towards some beautiful sandy island. The storm abated as the contraction passed. Charlie was born in a birthing pool in our kitchen, on 15 April 2002, weighing 6 lb 2 oz (2.8 kg). Everything went brilliantly, and I look back on it as an incredible experience.'

Case study – Lucy

Lucy had not practised yoga before she became pregnant, and chose to use some of the breathing practices during her labour: 'I found the Golden thread exhalations (p. 18) INVALUABLE! I used this breathing technique throughout my labour and it got me through. By focusing on my breath I was unaware of anything else around me and was really aware of my body and baby. I think it helped to keep me really calm and minimize the pain so I only needed to use gas and air for pain relief throughout. My baby daughter, Sophie Catherine was born at King's College Hospital, on 14 December 2006 weighing 7 lb 13 oz (3.5 kg).'

The different experiences described by Anna, Frankie, Jessamie and Lucy illustrate just how flexible and adaptable yoga practice can be during labour. There is no blueprint for a 'yoga birth'.

Teresa Arias, a south London midwife who has cared for many women who have attended yoga classes, comments:

> I think that one can tell, as a midwife, when someone has been to yoga for pregnancy classes for several reasons. Women, often for the first time, are encouraged to 'listen' and tune in to their bodies. This, I think, gives women confidence in themselves for birth and beyond. It helps them understand their bodies and reduces the fear factor. These women also seem more able to return to some sort of equilibrium at very challenging points in their labour when they are feeling panicky and losing their way.

Take heart from these stories, use the breath, movement and awareness practices to suit you, and never forget that birth is unpredictable, so a yogic attitude of open-hearted acceptance is your strongest ally.

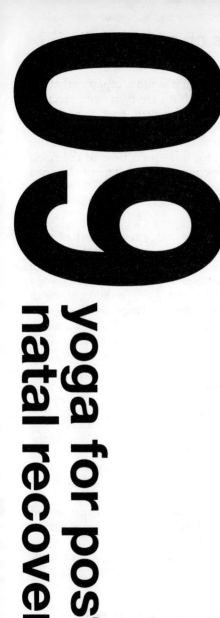

09

yoga for post-natal recovery

In this chapter you will learn:
- how yoga can help you adjust to motherhood and bond with your baby
- how yoga breath and pelvic floor practices can promote post-natal healing
- yoga programmes for different stages of post-natal recovery.

Yoga perspectives on post-natal recovery

The essential yogic attitudes of openness and acceptance that are so valuable during pregnancy and birth are even more precious after the birth of your baby. The immediate post-natal period can be a time of great elation, and also profound vulnerability and depression. It is a precious time for building the foundations of a relationship with the baby, but also a time of dramatic change and readjustment. Re-connecting to some of the yoga practices learnt during pregnancy provides a powerful system of holistic healing, and a comforting emotional link with life before birth, for both mother and baby.

In the first few days, or sometimes weeks, after the birth of your baby, yoga poses are not the most helpful aspect of yoga practice, and emphasis should be instead upon healing from inside out with breathing. As recovery progresses, however, yoga poses can be of great assistance in regaining stability, strength and vitality. This chapter provides guidance using yoga to promote post-natal recovery, and offers specific programmes appropriate to different stages of the post-natal period.

Post-natal challenges

In addition to the enormous emotional challenges of the adjustment to motherhood, common physical difficulties include lower back pain and weak abdominal muscles. Softness in the pelvic floor, piles, and sometimes injuries to the perineum following birth can make it feel as if there is no support for the base of the body, and it can be difficult to find a comfortable sitting position. Following caesarean birth, the weakness in the abdominal and pelvic area is exacerbated by the tenderness of wound healing. Feeding tiny babies can also cause stiff necks, shoulders and tightness in the upper back. The yoga programmes address all of these issues, offering a gentle but effective route to recovery.

Yoga breath and energy work for post-natal recovery

Along with the core breaths, many of the practices described in Chapters 03 and 04 can either be modified to promote effective post-natal recovery, or practised with a different perspective to gain specific post-natal benefits. For example, Golden thread exhalation (p. 18) is helpful to alleviate feelings of anxiety and panic that sometimes accompany the arrival of a baby; the calming effects of Breath balancing and Psychic alternate nostril breathing (pp. 154 and 156) can be very stabilizing and comforting during periods of volatile emotional swings, when your moods may alternate very rapidly. Further tips on the application of yoga breath in the post-natal period are given below:

Full yogic breath

This is an extremely helpful energizer. At times of exhaustion and desperation, just two or three rhythmic cycles of Full yogic breath (p. 13) can completely alter your state of mind and feeling of heart. Each phase of Full yogic breath brings its own benefits for you post-natally. Abdominal breathing is an effective and gentle way to regain tone in abdominal muscles, whilst chest breath encourages a more open feeling in the chest, relieving hunched back and shoulders from carrying and feeding infants. Remembering to 'sneak in' extra breath up to the collarbones provides a welcome boost of energy, especially when feeding small babies, and/or feeling exhausted as a result of sleep deprivation.

Ujjayi breath

Ujjayi (p. 16) is a useful soporific breath that can be especially helpful to settle into rest during and after breastfeeding. It brings about a state of deep quiet, and lowers blood pressure. Especially if it is done quite audibly, then it seems to be 'contagious', and its rhythmic sound can soothe babies and encourage them to drift off to sleep. Distressed babies, when held close to an Ujjayi-breathing mother, can hear the calming sound of the breath very clearly, because it is so much louder than the usual kind of breath. This can be a helpful soothing device in any situation where your baby is alarmed or upset.

Bhramari

Post-natally, the practice of bhramari (p. 151) can be a lifesaver. Babies usually find it deeply amusing, and its sound provides an instant, private retreat space for a stressed or exhausted mother.

Protective egg

This Protective egg technique (p. 152) works well for mothers and babies together. Your breath is an audible sound with which your baby can connect, whilst your mental focus creates the protective egg around you and your child. It is especially useful if your baby is alarmed, or if you are frightened and want to protect your baby from the feelings you are experiencing.

Entrainment breathing

Entrainment breathing (p. 157) is a versatile mothering tool to connect with babies and it is especially helpful as a calming practice. With tiny babies, close physical contact makes it possible to lead and pace their breath just from an awareness of its movement.

In addition to benefiting from the use of familiar pranayama learnt in pregnancy, post-natal recovery can also can be assisted by the Healing breath, specifically devised for post-natal women.

Healing breath with mula bandha

This relaxing breath returns along the path of the Birthing breath. It helps to resettle pelvic organs into a non-pregnant configuration, and provides gentle but energizing toning for the muscles of pelvic floor and abdomen. Notice that the instructions for this Healing breathing return to the usual yoga practice of lifting pelvic floor on exhale. This re-integration of breath and pelvic floor movements energizes and heals. It is valuable not only for women who birthed vaginally, but also for those who have had caesarean births, as it energizes and strengthens the abdomen and the lower back too.

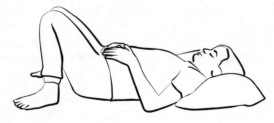

figure 9.1 Semi-supine

It is most effectively practised from semi-supine: soles of feet on floor, hip width apart, knees bent and touching.

1 Close eyes and establish a comfortable Full yogic breath.

2 Inhaling, let awareness flow up body from base of spine to crown of head.

3 Exhaling, let awareness flow down body from crown of head to base of spine.

4 As breath rhythm settles, notice soft hollowing of belly at end of exhalation, and how lower back eases down towards floor as belly 'sucks down'.

5 Let rhythmic cycle of breath draw awareness more towards exhalation, feeling that this hollowing of belly and lowering of lumbar spine to floor is building a connection to movement of pelvic floor. Inhale softly.

6 With next exhale, sense the drawing inwards and upwards of vagina towards cervix (mula bandha). If this movement does not happen spontaneously, then actively draw muscles in vaginal walls upwards and inward as you exhale.

7 Keep a gentle grip on this squeeze as you inhale.

8 As you next exhale, lift higher and squeeze tighter, feeling the action of these muscles quite high up inside.

9 Repeat this cycle once more.

10 On next inhalation, release hold on muscles, and return to two or three rhythmic breath cycles.

Tips

Work with awareness of pelvic floor and breath together, so that comfortable lengthening of breath is increasing strength in muscles. To start, tilt pelvis with breath, keeping buttocks on floor, lifting tailbone on exhale and arching lumbar spine a little away from floor on inhale. Use this process to connect with the hollowing of the belly (especially low down, close to pubic bone) and the lifting of pelvic floor. Once you are familiar with these feelings, then keep breath moving, but stop pelvic tilting, and develop awareness of internal movements.

The instructions above take you through one full round of Healing breath (i.e. two exhales and two inhales). Once you are comfortable with this, gradually increase the number of exhales which you make whilst the pelvic floor is lifted. When you are settled with a comfortable number of exhales per lift, stay with this, and alternate rounds of Healing breathing with a rhythmic cycle of Full yogic breath.

Yoga breath and sound for bonding with your baby

The familiar sounds and breathing rhythms that the baby heard in the womb throughout pregnancy can have an impressively soothing effect upon the child once it is born. Many mothers report with delight how readily their baby will settle to the gentle rhythm of their breath or the sounds they chanted during pregnancy. Tiny babies also love to rest on your chest or belly whilst slow rhythmic breathing continues: for this practice to be really comfortable for you, it is best to rest in semi-supine (p. 216). Let the gentle rise and fall of the body with the breath carry the baby along too.

Post-natal sonic massage

This transposes the mantras of Pre-natal sonic massage (p. 148) to the post-natal period, when the sounds create a pleasing continuity for babies who recall hearing them during their time in the womb. Even babies who only hear these sounds for the first time outside the womb find this sonic vibratory massage very soothing.

1 Lie your baby on a cushion on the floor, on his/her back or front, whichever he/she prefers.

2 Kneel down at your baby's feet and fold forwards, in Hare pose (p. 40) so that you rest easily over your baby and your mouth can come to touch his/her belly button. Hold his/her hands gently.

3 This is the base position, so ensure your back is long, not hunched up. Adjust distance from baby if necessary.

4 Exhaling, snuggle down towards your baby's navel and hum 'ramm' into centre of belly. Repeat mantra, either slowly or rapidly, for as long as you and your baby are enjoying it.

5 Then pause, adjust position and snuggle down so that your mouth is level with your baby's chest, and use the sounds of the Pre-natal sonic massage as follows: 'yamm' into centre of heart space on your baby's chest; 'hamm' into space between bottom of your baby's ear and top of their shoulder; and 'aumm' either into space between your baby's eyebrows, on forehead, or top of head. With each sound repeat either slowly or rapidly, for as long as you and your baby are enjoying it.

6 End by resting down by the side of your baby and practising the Full yogic breath.

Tips

If kneeling and folding forwards is not comfortable, adjust width of knees (wider is easier) and put cushions between heels and buttocks, or lay on your front with legs straight out behind, and weight of upper body supported on elbows.

Yoga meditation and relaxation for post-natal recovery

Comforting, re-energizing and deeply restorative, all the yoga meditations and relaxations described in Chapters 05 and 06 are especially helpful post-natally. The presence of your baby will change your experience of the practices, and part of their benefit is to help you understand and accept these differences. In particular, the Heart/womb breath, mudra and meditation (pp. 145 and 163) offer powerful reconnection with the changed energy of the uterus. Yoga nidra is also a particularly useful practice at this time. Either listen to the CD (**Audio CD track 5**), replacing inner awareness of the baby within the womb with an appreciation of the baby by your side or in your arms, or else use the written outline (p. 166) to create your own practice. It can be helpful to adopt a new sankalpa to encourage post-natal recovery.

One of the most valuable applications of yoga awareness to embrace the changes of the post-natal period is the Feeding meditation described below.

Feeding breath meditation

Audio CD track 6

This is a specific post-natal version of Inner silence meditation (p. 168) that works equally well whether you are breast or bottle-feeding your baby. It uses breath and sensory awareness to create calm and receptivity. Full instructions for the basic practice are given in Chapter 06, but Audio CD track 6 and the instructions below also include particular guidance for sensory awareness of your feeding baby.

1 Sit or lie in a position in which you can comfortably feed your baby.

2 Be generous with supports. Have as many pillows, blankets, cushions and props as you need to get really comfortable.

3 Hold your baby in such a way that he/she can feed easily, and that your shoulders, neck and arms are completely relaxed.

4 As you settle and the baby gets into the feed, watch your rhythmic breath cycle and follow the instructions on Audio CD track 6, or page 168, including the baby-specific guidance below.

5 Notice especially that when you exhale awareness into the sense of hearing, you are aware of the sound of the baby's breath, and the sound of the baby's feeding.

6 When you exhale awareness into the sense of touch, feel the warmth of the baby close to you and notice the different temperature of your skin where the baby is in close contact, in comparison to the skin on other parts of your body.

7 When you exhale awareness into the sense of smell, notice the smell of the baby, or the milk, or the smell of the baby's clothes.

8 After you have brought your attention to each sense, and returned to the sense of hearing, notice the sounds of the baby's feeding and breathing and follow the instructions (p. 169–170) to conclude the practice.

Tips

You can continue this meditation for the whole duration of a feed, or you can do it very swiftly just at the start and then simply rest with breath awareness for the remainder of the feed.

Yoga postures for post-natal recovery

Whereas much of the emphasis in pregnancy yoga postures is on opening and softening to create space for the bump, yoga for effective post-natal recovery focuses on stabilizing and strengthening. Most of the poses described in Chapter 03 should now be done with a narrower stance, and it is wise to avoid wide-legged stances (such as Warrior or squat-based poses) until pelvis and lower back feel more secure.

To counteract the hunched chest, stiff neck and shoulders that are often experienced post-natally, the Earthed seated flow is ideal (p. 181). All the healing sequences for relief from pain or discomfort (pp. 183–7) can also be helpful post-natally, if undertaken with certain precautions.

Cautions

Avoid standing practices until at least three weeks after birth, and then stand with feet much narrower than before, and replace pelvic floor practices for pregnancy with Healing breath (p. 216). Of these healing sequences, the ones for relief of lower back pain (p. 183), management of pelvic pain (p. 184), and for exhaustion (p. 188) are likely to be the most useful.

Post-natal yoga programmes

This section offers three basic programmes for post-natal recovery starting immediately after the birth of your baby, including caesarean birth. Each session can be adapted or extended to run from 5 to 20 minutes. All postures and breaths are described in previous chapters, except for those for which new illustrations are provided. Modifications of pregnancy yoga practices are also given.

Nurture

Suitable for immediate postpartum and during the first eight weeks, or any time when you feel more tired then usual. It is also an ideal programme from which to draw closing practices for yoga sessions done at later stages of post-natal recovery.

Have your baby by your side, or resting on your belly.

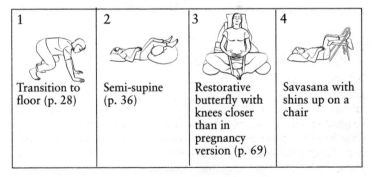

1	2	3	4
Transition to floor (p. 28)	Semi-supine (p. 36)	Restorative butterfly with knees closer than in pregnancy version (p. 69)	Savasana with shins up on a chair

Rest for as long as time permits in any of the above poses, whilst practising the below breath and awareness practices:

- Healing breath with Mula bandha (p. 216)
- Yoga Nidra with Sankalpa (p. 166)
- Feeding meditation (Audio CD track 6)

Stabilize

The physical aim of this programme is to stabilize the pelvis and lower back. Emotionally, the sound work promotes a sense of security and calm. It is suitable from 4 to 6 weeks post-natally right through the first year and beyond. It also provides a useful set of practices to maintain awareness of the need for physical and emotional stability, especially at times of accelerated change, for example, if you are returning to paid employment, or if your baby is making a major developmental leap such as weaning, or learning to sit up or crawl. With all the postures, use Healing breath with pelvic floor lift on exhale.

Cautions

Avoid pelvic lifts until six weeks after caesarean birth.

1	2	3	4
Transition to floor (p. 28)	Semi-supine (p. 216) Healing breath (p. 216) followed by pelvic tilting	Cat with your baby underneath you. Focus on pelvic floor lift and abdominial strength on exhale. Pelvic tilts and circles (p. 74)	Flowing hare-to cat swoop (p. 42)
5	6	7	8
Tiger part one (p. 48)	Hare pose for Postnatal sonic (p. 40)	Rest in semi-supine (p. 216) Sound releases in relaxation and/or natural soundings to release (p. 147)	Legs on chair (p. 221)

To stabilize the pelvis after pregnancy, it is crucial to emphasize support from buttock muscles, squeezing tight to ascertain their strength, and working with rhythmic squeezes and releases on pelvic tilts to build this strength. Move from tilts, to gentle rolls and lifts. Always lift and lower on exhale to engage effect of the Healing breath pelvic floor lift. To promote stability move knees closer together, placing a block between them, squeezing tight to hold it in place as you tilt and lift the pelvis.

Restore vitality

These are the practices to use at 8 to 12 weeks, or whenever you feel secure enough to move with a little more energy. This may be earlier than eight weeks, depending upon your level of fitness before the birth, the nature of the birth and the pace of your post-natal recovery experience.

Cautions

Throughout this sequence, bring attention to support from buttocks, abdominals and pelvic floor.

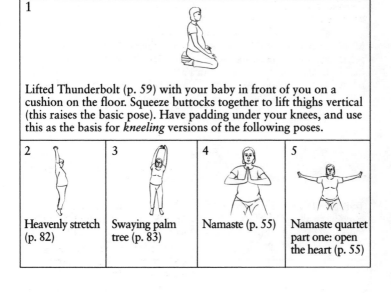

1
Lifted Thunderbolt (p. 59) with your baby in front of you on a cushion on the floor. Squeeze buttocks together to lift thighs vertical (this raises the basic pose). Have padding under your knees, and use this as the basis for *kneeling* versions of the following poses.

2	3	4	5
Heavenly stretch (p. 82)	Swaying palm tree (p. 83)	Namaste (p. 55)	Namaste quartet part one: open the heart (p. 55)

6	7	8	9
Namaste quartet part two: life the spirits (p. 56)	Namaste quartet part three: reach with ease (p. 56)	Namaste quartet part four: build vitality (p. 57)	Cat inhale and exhale, three repetitions (p. 39)

10	11		
Flowing hare-to cat swoop inhale and exhale, three repetitions (p. 42)	Stick pose (p. 53) Bring legs and ankles together, sitting on block with your baby by your side or on your lap. Use this as a basis for Energy freeing series for feet and arms (p. 120–133). Do one arm at a time if you need to hold your baby steady.		

12	13
Mountain pose against the wall using pelvic tilts, rocks, scoops and circles (p. 81), holding your baby close with relaxed neck and shoulders. Keep knees and ankles together.	Chair against wall, up to seven rounds of breath (p. 99). Slide up and down wall a little way, holding your baby close with relaxed neck and shoulders. Keep knees and ankles together.

14	15	
Transition from standing to all fours (p. 28)	Transition from all fours and down to floor (p. 30)	To close sequence, Yoga Nidra (p. 166). Audio CD track 5 and/or feeding meditation (p. 219) Audio CD track 6.

Yoga in everyday life

Initially, it is best to practice Healing breath in semi-supine (p. 216). But once you are comfortable with it, it works well sitting too. Done gently, to the natural rhythm of the Full yogic breath cycle, it makes a great accompaniment to feeding a baby. As you sit to nourish the infant, then you are also nourishing, healing and energizing yourself from within.

Once you have practised the Healing breath in resting and sitting positions, then it is easy to transpose its benefits to everyday life. The awareness of the lifted mula bandha on the exhale is especially useful when lifting and carrying babies. Often the lower back pain experienced by post-natal mothers is a combined result of weakened pelvic floor and abdominal muscles, exacerbated by unconsciously damaging lifting techniques. Since your little baby will soon grow heavier, and you will be constantly picking her up and putting her down, anything that brings conscious support into the process is going to minimize possible injury and discomfort. For example, if you are sitting on the floor and aiming to lift your baby as you come up to standing, then let Healing breath begins as you first hold your baby. Exhale to contact the lift in your pelvic floor, inhale as you ready yourself to stand (still keeping pelvic floor lifted), and then exhale again as you come to your feet, holding pelvic floor, lift as you raise up with your baby in your arms. 'Lift yourself before you lift your child' is the affirmation to bear in mind as you transpose the Healing breath into the lifting breath for everyday use.

glossary

The following is a selection of terms used in this book, gathered here for quick reference. For more information on each of them, please refer to the relevant index entry.

Agni Fire element.

Akasha Ether element, or the space in which all other elements exist.

Apana vayu Downward movement of energy, from the navel to the perineum

Apas Water element.

Asana Literally meaning 'seat', but usually understood as yoga postures.

Ayurveda Indian medical system that shares a philosophical framework with yoga.

Chakras Literally 'wheel': spinning energy centres in the pranic body.

Coccyx The 'tailbone', fused to the bottom of the sacrum, but mobile enough during pregnancy to allow it to move backwards to create more space for birth of baby.

Diaphragm The respiratory diaphragm is a musculo-tendinous sheet that divides the contents of the abdominal cavity (including the stomach, intestines, liver and kidneys) from the contents of the thoracic cavity (the heart and lungs). It consists of a central tendinous area surrounded by skeletal muscle fibres that run from the edges of a central tendon to attach to the sides of the ribs and the spine.

Hridaya Spiritual heart.

Ilium Broad, curved bone at side of pelvis, one on either side. Iliac crests are felt at the widest point of the hips.

Mudra Psycho-neural gestures that alter the flow of energy in the body-mind. They include hasta mudras, which are principally finger locks and hand gestures, pelvic floor movements, and full-body mudras which involve posture, breath and awareness.

Nadis Energy channels.

Oedema Swelling due to excess fluid in the body.

Optimal foetal positioning The best position for the baby in the womb to facilitate an easier birth.

Pelvic floor The hammock of muscles at the bottom of the pelvis, in which are located sphincters, or muscular locks controlling the function of the urethra (opening from bladder to release urine), anus (opening from bowel to release faeces) and vagina (opening from womb to release baby).

Pelvis Bony ring at base of spine, commonly referred to as the 'hips'. It is formed of three bones: at the back is the sacrum, with the coccyx attached, and at the sides are the two ilium bones. During pregnancy, the joints between these bones become more mobile.

Perineum Generally understood as the pelvic floor, sometimes more specifically used to refer to the area between vagina and anus.

Placenta The baby's 'life support' system, the interface through which blood and nutrients from the mother are filtered to the unborn child in the womb.

Prana Vital energy or life force.

Pranayama Literally translated as the 'expansion of the life force', this is usually understood as any yoga practices, especially breathing techniques, that work with the energy body.

Prithvi Earth element.

Pubic symphysis dysfunction (PSD or SPD) Pain due to separation and/or movement, and/or inflammation of the pubic symphysis.

Pubic symphysis Joint between two ilium bones, at the front of the pelvis.

Sacroiliac joint Joint between sacrum and ilium in the back of the pelvis.

Sacrum Flat bone at the back of the pelvis.

Shakti bandha Energy block releasing pose.

Shunya Purification.

Surya Sun.

Swara Flow of breath in the nostrils.

Tattva Elements.

Trimester One-third of the length of full term pregnancy.

Upanisads Spiritual and philosophical texts at the end of the Vedas, Hindu scriptures.

Uterus Womb.

Vayu Air element.

Vertebrae Bones of the spine.

taking it further

Books

There are so many books about yoga, pregnancy and birth that it can be hard to know where to start. This list guides you to some of the most useful texts, and outlines what you can expect to learn from them.

Baker, Jeannine Parvati. 1974 (Silver Anniversary 3rd edition 2001). *Pre-natal Yoga and Natural Childbirth*. North Atlantic Books, Berkeley CA.

This is where it all started, the first book to bring together the ideas of yoga and pregnancy. A visionary voice, way ahead of her time, the late Parvati Baker's book is full of inspiring birth stories and spiritual explorations.

Balaskas, Janet. 1994. *Preparing for Birth with Yoga*. Element, London.

A key text in the development of pregnancy yoga, by the founder of the Active Birth movement. Its tone and approach are rooted in the north London women's yoga group that pioneered yoga for pregnancy as a part of a successful campaign challenging hospital birthing protocols in the 1980s.

Chiarelli, Pauline. *Women's Waterworks*. Neem Press.

An invaluable practical guide to the female pelvic floor, by a physiotherapist and continence advisor. A free e-book version is available to download at **www.womenswaterworks.com**

Dinsmore-Tuli, Uma. 2006. *Mother's Breath: a definitive guide to yoga breathing, sound and awareness practices during pregnancy, birth, post-natal recovery and mothering*. Sitaram and Sons. London.

The ideal companion to *Teach Yourself Yoga for Pregnancy and Birth,* this is the most comprehensive guide to every aspect of yoga breath and awareness for mothers and expectant mothers. Detailed instructions and plenty of lively personal testimony from women who have used these practices.

England, Pam & Horowitz, Rob. 1998. *Birthing from Within: An Extra-ordinary guide to Childbirth Preparation*. Partera Press: Albuquerque, New Mexico.

A remarkably useful array of multi-sensory methods to preparing for birth, including birth art, pain coping techniques, ritual and singing, by the founder of the Birthing from Within approach.

Freedman, Françoise. 2004. *Yoga for Pregnancy, birth and beyond*. Dorling Kindersley. London.

A beautiful exposition of the Birthlight approach to yoga in pregnancy. Some helpful ideas and creative asanas for pregnancy and post-natal recovery, all gorgeously photographed.

Gaskin, Ina May. 1977 [1990]. *Spiritual Midwifery*. The Book Publishing Company: Summertown, Tennessee.

A classic text full of inspiring stories that transform expectations about birth.

Kitzinger, Sheila. 2003. *The New pregnancy and childbirth: choices and challenges*. Dorling Kindersely. London.

User-friendly guide, packed with information, clear diagrams and sensible suggestions.

Lasater, Judith Hanson. 2000. *Living your yoga: finding the spiritual in everyday life*. Rodmell Press: Berkeley, California.

Full of encouraging references to family life and the incorporation of yoga into daily experience.

Motha, Gowri. 2004. *Gentle Birth Method*. Thorsons: London.

A detailed programme designed by the obstetrician who pioneered waterbirth in the UK. Including diet, exercise and complementary therapies, plus birth stories and self-hypnosis in labour.

Romm, Aviva Jill. 2002. *Natural Health After Birth: the complete guide to postpartum wellness*. Healing Arts Press, Rochester Vermont.

A friendly, accessible holistic guide to post-natal recovery, including yoga, herbal remedies and tasty recipes.

Stadlen, Naomi. 2004. *What Mothers Do, especially when it looks like nothing*. Piatkus. London.

Absolutely indispensable for all new mothers. A thoughtful and perceptive account of mothering by an existential psychotherapist, mother and breastfeeding counsellor. A kind, compassionate and open-hearted book, full of insight.

Sutton, Jean. 2000. *Let Birth Be Born Again.* Birth Concepts. London.

Complete explanation of theory and practice of optimal foetal positioning by one of its most passionate advocates.

Teasdill Wendy. 2000. *Yoga for Pregnancy.* Gaia. London.

An engaging and holistic illustrated guide, with practices for every stage of pregnancy and the immediate post-natal period, including practical applications of yoga philosophy.

Verny, Thomas, with Kelly, John. 1981. *The Secret Life of the Unborn Child.* Warner. London.

A fascinating summary of research, including a chapter on 'the first year' in utero and post-natally.

Special recommendation

Mother's Breath is warmly recommended if you would like to know more about yoga breath, sound and awareness practices for pregnancy, childbirth, post-natal recovery and mothering. As well as practical instructions and testimonies, it includes further detailed technical information for health professionals, yoga teachers and practitioners. In addition to this very useful book, audio CDs and DVDs can be helpful resources to continue your yoga in pregnancy, providing further instruction and motivation for home sessions.

The sample tracks provided on the CD in this book are extracts from the following audio CDs, all of which give you a range of safe and appropriate breath, sound, relaxation and mediation practices for pregnancy. For further instruction in asana, see instead the DVD listing which follows.

Mother's Breath and all the following resources, as well as a complete range of high quality yoga props and equipment including mats, blocks and balls, are available by mail order from:

Yogamatters
32 Clarendon Road
London N8 0D
Tel: (+44) [0]20 8888 8588
Fax: (+44) [0]20 8888 0623
E-mail: www.yogamatters.com.

For bulk trade orders of *Mother's Breath* and other Sitaram Products, please contact the publishers, Sitaram and Sons: www.sitaram.org or (+44) [0]20 8678 0054.

Audio CDs

Mother's Breath triple CD set

A unique resource, providing clear guidance for all the breath, sound, awareness and pelvic floor techniques described in the *Mother's Breath* book. In addition to the sample tracks on the CD that comes with this book, there are 31 different techniques on three separate 60-minute discs for pregnancy and post-natal recovery, plus a 'mother's voice' disc which is appropriate for pre- and post-natal practice.

Yoga Birth 1

Deeply soothing, nurturing yoga for pregnant women: gentle stretches, relaxation, breathing practices to energize and calm including breaths for use in labour. In addition to the two sample tracks on the CD included with this book, there is also a range of breath work and a deep relaxation practice (yoga nidra) with a breathing sequence to take you through contractions to the birth of your baby. 70 minutes.

Yoga babies Songs for Yoga Babies and Relaxation for Mums

Audio guidance recorded live in a class of mothers and babies, with action songs and rhymes to sing with your baby whilst you do yoga together. Words and actions all on the inside cover. In addition to the Feeding meditation on the CD included with this book, tracks include Post-natal sonic massage and a deep relaxation for mums. 70 minutes.

Simply Calm

70 minutes of breath, visualization and deep relaxation for stress relief, including yoga nidra. Simple but profoundly restful techniques designed to bring about a state of calm. Each practice can be done independently, or as a complete session. Although not specifically aimed at pregnant women, all practices are safe for use during pregnancy, and can be very useful for birth companions.

DVDs

Sitaram Mother Nurture: Yoga for pregnancy, yoga for birth and yoga for post-natal recovery with babies. DVD triple set.

The recommended audio visual companion to this book. Fully integrated programme of over 25 practices across three 60-minute DVDs: the first for all stages of pregnancy, the second for birth preparation (with and without a partner), and the third for practice with your baby up to eight months. Breath, movement, sound practices and deep relaxation in flowing sequences.

Wendy Teasdill's *Yoga for Pregnancy and Childbirth* and *Yoga for Post-natal Vitality*.

Two separate DVDs of yoga exercises and relaxation techniques to help women throughout pregnancy achieve a greater sense of well-being and confidence.

Little Gems Simple Yoga for Pregnancy, Simple Yoga for Birth and *Simple Post-natal Yoga*

Three individual, hour long DVDs suitable for women who have never practiced yoga before. Clear instructions emphasizing the importance of stretching, breathing techniques and relaxation.

Yoga training and classes

Many committed yoga practitioners and teachers first came to yoga during pregnancy. If you want to learn more about the yoga teachings upon which this book is founded, then the following books will be of interest:

Swami Satyananda Sarswati. 1996. *Asana, Pranayama, Mudra, Bandha*. Bihar School of Yoga, Munger, Bihar, India.

A comprehensive guide to all aspects of yoga, including breath, gesture, energy locks, esoteric anatomy, yoga psychology and therapeutic applications.

Mukunda Stiles. 2000. *Structural Yoga Therapy*. Weiser, United States.

Thorough and thoughtful guidance on yoga for holistic health. Includes detailed information about standard range of motion and yoga asana. Also www.yogatherapycenter.org: for case studies by structural yoga therapists, and answers to many questions about appropriate yoga therapeutic responses.

Yoga for pregnancy training

Because there are a number of different organizations offering training in pregnancy yoga, it can sometimes be confusing or difficult to identify a suitable local teacher. You may need to consult the registers of all of the training bodies listed below to discover the classes nearest to you.

If you are interested in training as a yoga for pregnancy or post-natal recovery teacher, or if you want to know more about the training of a particular teacher, then it is wisest to obtain the syllabus for each of the courses described below, and compare it with what is on offer elsewhere, since there are some overlaps, but also differences in approach.

Not all teachers/trainers offering yoga for pregnancy classes/courses are fully qualified general yoga teachers with skills or interest in the complete range of yoga practices. This may not be an issue if you are new to yoga, but if you are looking for depth of guidance and informed understanding of a range of yoga techniques such as the ones described in this book, then ask the prospective teacher/trainer about their qualifications and experience first.

Sitaram Partnership

Tel:+ 44 (0)208 678 0054
E-mail:www.sitaram.org
Courses: pregnancy yoga, post-natal yoga and early years yoga.

Training and classes offered by the author, and teachers trained in the methods described in this book.

Life centre education

Tel: +44 (0)208 826 4726
E-mail: www.thelifecentre.org
Courses: pregnancy yoga, post-natal yoga, early years yoga, yoga therapy foundation and diploma.

Pre-requisites: general yoga teacher training qualification from any tradition (either completed or a minimum of 6 months in progress). Emphasis upon integrated and restorative practice including breath, sound, Mudra, movement, deep relaxation, meditation and awareness techniques. Also, introductory days in the safe integration of pregnant and post-natal students in general yoga classes.

British Wheel of Yoga

E-mail: www.bwy.org.uk
Tel: Central Office 01529 30685

Courses: pregnancy yoga and post-natal yoga modules (see also Sitaram partnership above).

Pre-requisites: General yoga teacher training diploma for pregnancy yoga module and for post-natal yoga (see above).

Birthlight

E-mail: www.birthlight.com
Tel: 0771 458 6153

Courses: perinatal yoga, baby yoga and a range of other yoga-based practices for mothers and babies, including aqua yoga.

Pre-requisites: for perinatal yoga, a general yoga teacher training qualification. For all other courses no previous yoga experience is required.

Yogabirth

E-mail: www.yogabirth.co.uk
Tel: 0208 769 3613
Courses: pregnancy yoga

Prerequisite: open to all yoga teachers and serious practitioners of yoga. A probationary year working with a mentor follows the course and precedes qualification.

Active Birth

E-mail: www.activebirthcentre.com
Tel: 020 7281 6760
Courses: active birth, yoga for pregnancy and post-natal yoga.

Prerequisite: No yoga qualifications required.

Other useful contacts

Birthing From Within

For classes and training in birth preparation.

E-mail: www.birthingfromwithin.com

National Childbirth Trust

E-mail: www.nct.org.uk

For local antenatal classes, post-natal support, breastfeeding counselling and information on pregnancy, childbirth, breastfeeding and parenthood.

Pelvic partnership

E-mail: www.pelvicpartnership.org.uk

Information and support for women with pelvic pain.

Post-natal illness

E-mail: www.pni.org.uk

Support and information for women with post-natal depression.

See also www.mind.org.uk for useful pamphlets and local support networks.

SANDS

E-mail: www.uk-sands.org

For support and information about stillbirth and neonatal death.

teach yourself ®

From Advanced Sudoku to Zulu, you'll find everything you need in the **teach yourself** range, in books, on CD and on DVD.

Visit **www.teachyourself.co.uk** for more details.

Advanced Sudoku and Kakuro
Afrikaans
Alexander Technique
Algebra
Ancient Greek
Applied Psychology
Arabic
Arabic Conversation
Aromatherapy
Art History
Astrology
Astronomy
AutoCAD 2004
AutoCAD 2007
Ayurveda
Baby Massage and Yoga
Baby Signing
Baby Sleep
Bach Flower Remedies
Backgammon
Ballroom Dancing
Basic Accounting
Basic Computer Skills
Basic Mathematics
Beauty
Beekeeping
Beginner's Arabic Script
Beginner's Chinese Script
Beginner's Dutch

Beginner's French
Beginner's German
Beginner's Greek
Beginner's Greek Script
Beginner's Hindi
Beginner's Hindi Script
Beginner's Italian
Beginner's Japanese
Beginner's Japanese Script
Beginner's Latin
Beginner's Mandarin Chinese
Beginner's Portuguese
Beginner's Russian
Beginner's Russian Script
Beginner's Spanish
Beginner's Turkish
Beginner's Urdu Script
Bengali
Better Bridge
Better Chess
Better Driving
Better Handwriting
Biblical Hebrew
Biology
Birdwatching
Blogging
Body Language
Book Keeping
Brazilian Portuguese

Bridge
British Citizenship Test, The
British Empire, The
British Monarchy from Henry VIII, The
Buddhism
Bulgarian
Bulgarian Conversation
Business French
Business Plans
Business Spanish
Business Studies
C++
Calculus
Calligraphy
Cantonese
Caravanning
Car Buying and Maintenance
Card Games
Catalan
Chess
Chi Kung
Chinese Medicine
Christianity
Classical Music
Coaching
Cold War, The
Collecting
Computing for the Over 50s
Consulting
Copywriting
Correct English
Counselling
Creative Writing
Cricket
Croatian
Crystal Healing
CVs
Czech
Danish
Decluttering
Desktop Publishing
Detox
Digital Home Movie Making
Digital Photography
Dog Training

Drawing
Dream Interpretation
Dutch
Dutch Conversation
Dutch Dictionary
Dutch Grammar
Eastern Philosophy
Electronics
English as a Foreign Language
English Grammar
English Grammar as a Foreign Language
Entrepreneurship
Estonian
Ethics
Excel 2003
Feng Shui
Film Making
Film Studies
Finance for Non-Financial Managers
Finnish
First World War, The
Fitness
Flash 8
Flash MX
Flexible Working
Flirting
Flower Arranging
Franchising
French
French Conversation
French Dictionary
French for Homebuyers
French Grammar
French Phrasebook
French Starter Kit
French Verbs
French Vocabulary
Freud
Gaelic
Gaelic Conversation
Gaelic Dictionary
Gardening
Genetics
Geology

German
German Conversation
German Grammar
German Phrasebook
German Starter Kit
German Vocabulary
Globalization
Go
Golf
Good Study Skills
Great Sex
Green Parenting
Greek
Greek Conversation
Greek Phrasebook
Growing Your Business
Guitar
Gulf Arabic
Hand Reflexology
Hausa
Herbal Medicine
Hieroglyphics
Hindi
Hindi Conversation
Hinduism
History of Ireland, The
Home PC Maintenance and
  Networking
How to DJ
How to Run a Marathon
How to Win at Casino Games
How to Win at Horse Racing
How to Win at Online Gambling
How to Win at Poker
How to Write a Blockbuster
Human Anatomy & Physiology
Hungarian
Icelandic
Improve Your French
Improve Your German
Improve Your Italian
Improve Your Spanish
Improving Your Employability
Indian Head Massage
Indonesian
Instant French

Instant German
Instant Greek
Instant Italian
Instant Japanese
Instant Portuguese
Instant Russian
Instant Spanish
Internet, The
Irish
Irish Conversation
Irish Grammar
Islam
Israeli-Palestinian Conflict, The
Italian
Italian Conversation
Italian for Homebuyers
Italian Grammar
Italian Phrasebook
Italian Starter Kit
Italian Verbs
Italian Vocabulary
Japanese
Japanese Conversation
Java
JavaScript
Jazz
Jewellery Making
Judaism
Jung
Kama Sutra, The
Keeping Aquarium Fish
Keeping Pigs
Keeping Poultry
Keeping a Rabbit
Knitting
Korean
Latin
Latin American Spanish
Latin Dictionary
Latin Grammar
Letter Writing Skills
Life at 50: For Men
Life at 50: For Women
Life Coaching
Linguistics
LINUX

Lithuanian
Magic
Mahjong
Malay
Managing Stress
Managing Your Own Career
Mandarin Chinese
Mandarin Chinese Conversation
Marketing
Marx
Massage
Mathematics
Meditation
Middle East Since 1945, The
Modern China
Modern Hebrew
Modern Persian
Mosaics
Music Theory
Mussolini's Italy
Nazi Germany
Negotiating
Nepali
New Testament Greek
NLP
Norwegian
Norwegian Conversation
Old English
One-Day French
One-Day French – the DVD
One-Day German
One-Day Greek
One-Day Italian
One-Day Polish
One-Day Portuguese
One-Day Spanish
One-Day Spanish – the DVD
One-Day Turkish
Origami
Owning a Cat
Owning a Horse
Panjabi
PC Networking for Small
   Businesses
Personal Safety and Self Defence
Philosophy

Philosophy of Mind
Philosophy of Religion
Phone French
Phone German
Phone Italian
Phone Japanese
Phone Mandarin Chinese
Phone Spanish
Photography
Photoshop
PHP with MySQL
Physics
Piano
Pilates
Planning Your Wedding
Polish
Polish Conversation
Politics
Portuguese
Portuguese Conversation
Portuguese for Homebuyers
Portuguese Grammar
Portuguese Phrasebook
Postmodernism
Pottery
PowerPoint 2003
PR
Project Management
Psychology
Quick Fix French Grammar
Quick Fix German Grammar
Quick Fix Italian Grammar
Quick Fix Spanish Grammar
Quick Fix: Access 2002
Quick Fix: Excel 2000
Quick Fix: Excel 2002
Quick Fix: HTML
Quick Fix: Windows XP
Quick Fix: Word
Quilting
Recruitment
Reflexology
Reiki
Relaxation
Retaining Staff
Romanian

Running Your Own Business
Russian
Russian Conversation
Russian Grammar
Sage Line 50
Sanskrit
Screenwriting
Second World War, The
Serbian
Setting Up a Small Business
Shorthand Pitman 2000
Sikhism
Singing
Slovene
Small Business Accounting
Small Business Health Check
Songwriting
Spanish
Spanish Conversation
Spanish Dictionary
Spanish for Homebuyers
Spanish Grammar
Spanish Phrasebook
Spanish Starter Kit
Spanish Verbs
Spanish Vocabulary
Speaking On Special Occasions
Speed Reading
Stalin's Russia
Stand Up Comedy
Statistics
Stop Smoking
Sudoku
Swahili
Swahili Dictionary
Swedish
Swedish Conversation
Tagalog
Tai Chi
Tantric Sex
Tap Dancing
Teaching English as a Foreign
    Language
Teams & Team Working
Thai
Thai Conversation

Theatre
Time Management
Tracing Your Family History
Training
Travel Writing
Trigonometry
Turkish
Turkish Conversation
Twentieth Century USA
Typing
Ukrainian
Understanding Tax for Small
    Businesses
Understanding Terrorism
Urdu
Vietnamese
Visual Basic
Volcanoes, Earthquakes and
    Tsunamis
Watercolour Painting
Weight Control through Diet &
    Exercise
Welsh
Welsh Conversation
Welsh Dictionary
Welsh Grammar
Wills & Probate
Windows XP
Wine Tasting
Winning at Job Interviews
Word 2003
World Faiths
Writing Crime Fiction
Writing for Children
Writing for Magazines
Writing a Novel
Writing a Play
Writing Poetry
Xhosa
Yiddish
Yoga
Your Wedding
Zen
Zulu

teach yourself

baby massage and yoga
anita epple and pauline carpenter

- Would you like to improve your baby's wellbeing?
- Do you want to deepen your parent–child bond?
- Do you need basic instructions for gentle massage and yoga exercises?

Baby Massage and Yoga will introduce you and your child to the benefits of massage and to some simple yoga stretches. The sensible, step-by-step advice and techniques are designed to help you deepen both your bond and your child's development at every level.

Anita Epple and **Pauline Carpenter** are fully qualified infant Massage Teachers, and the co-directors of Touch-Learn, a training organisation that trains infant Massage Teachers.